NAUTI GIRL

Navigating my naked truth
from trauma to triumph

STEPHANIE
KRAEMER

ISBN: 978-1-960136-14-5

Disclaimer

Trigger warnings: I reference trauma in this memoir, both big T or small t. Most people associate trauma with larger issues, but there is no right or wrong for what someone is triggered by, or how it influences their life. Trauma can present itself differently for everyone, ranging from email communication to bullying to death. Even the word triggered, by nature, can feel very provoking at times.

Writing is my creative expression for healing. It externalizes what I've been carrying on the inside. The physical act of putting words on a page is freeing, reducing the space trauma has held in my life. This is not a "victim's account" of the past. Every word has been a step forward in my journey. And each step has connected me with my inner child to feel more empowered. My hope is that this book opens an avenue for you to feel the same.

These are my recollections, and might differ from others perspectives.

Except for my husband, I've replaced all names and done my best to obscure all identities for reasons that will become clear.

Water is the underlying current of the book, because we are primarily made of water. It flows through us, around us, and represents cleansing and healing. Its powerful essence helps connect us to something bigger than ourselves, forming deep feelings of renewal and purpose. Water-themed references, along with innuendo flirting, flow throughout these pages.

As you will discover, I have the heart and mouth of a sailor. Some things I share might feel activating, controversial, or even offensive, but I refuse to apologize for my truth.

I've spent a lot of my life thinking I was drowning...

Dedication

To my former self, who needed a hero, so that's what she became.

And to all of you feeling adrift, who have a hero inside you too.

I'm grateful you picked up this book! It serves as a reminder to fearlessly show up for life every day.

Thank you for the opportunity to explore the darkness, be vulnerable, and shift bravely into the light. These writings are not only dedicated to my inner child, but to you, too.

This book is my gift.

This book is my naked truth.

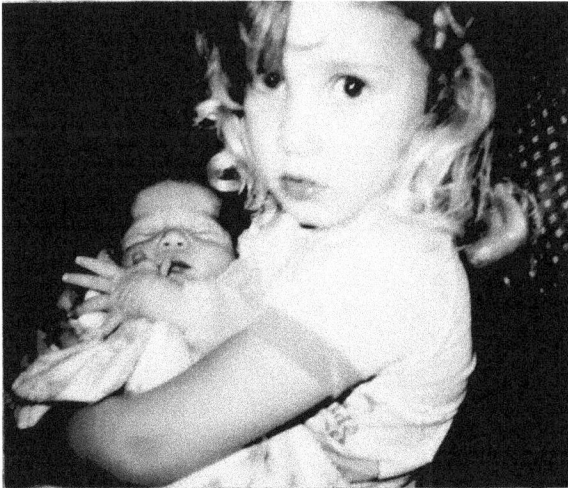

Prologue

"The cure for anything is salt water; sweat, tears and the sea. Salt water heals physical wounds, sweat heals infections, tears heal mental wounds, and the sea can heal everything." —Isak Dinesen

---

I don't like to brag, but I've experienced a lot of trauma.

While some people show their scars on the outside, others like myself wear their wounds on the inside.

Trauma can feel like a hole ripped through the very fabric of your being. And even after you do all these things to heal, the hole seems to shrink, yet leaves behind jagged edges. Many feel like a piece of them will always be missing. But what if I told you that nothing is ever missing?

Every part, good or bad, will always be there with you. No experience, regardless of how ugly it was, disappears. It simply gets buried. For where there was deep trauma, there was also great love.

Do not be ashamed of the trauma.
Do not judge it.
Do not wish it away.
Do not rush it.

Keep going. That's all you really have to do.
Slow is fine.
Crawling is fine.

But, I encourage you to acknowledge it.
Lean into it.
Listen to it.

Feel it. Really feel it.
Sit with it.

When I sat down to write this book, I had no idea where to begin. But there I was, naked; truth dripping from the seams of my soul.

Table of Contents

INTRODUCTION
The Secret of the Sea

"Would you learn the secret of the sea? Only those who brave its dangers, comprehend its mystery!"
—Henry Wadsworth Longfellow

"You should really write a book, Steph." I can't tell you how many times I heard these words throughout my life. And they were right! While this is incredibly challenging to write, I know it's critical to my own healing journey.

The birth of this book has been a labor of love, an attempt to purge the "disease to please" that grew from my silence and lack of self-worth. For years, my mind and body have ached under the weight of others' burdens. My freedom lives in these pages.

A compilation of personal stories, reflections, and suggested activities, my writing exposes hidden parts of me confirmed through years of journaling and experience. My writing focuses on courageously showing up for ourselves every day, sharing strategies which supported me along the way.

My hope is that, together, we reframe trauma to create energy and space for our own healing.

This book isn't about guaranteeing trauma recovery or following an expert's 10-step process to "fix ourselves." In fact, I don't believe anyone ever truly "recovers" from trauma - and honestly, it would be a shame if we did. Trauma shapes us, connects us, and gives us the profound ability to relate to others. So, instead of chasing recovery, I believe we can learn to embrace the gifts that come from our pain.

This book is my memoir of vulnerability. If sharing it even helps one person, then I am happy I put it out to the masses.

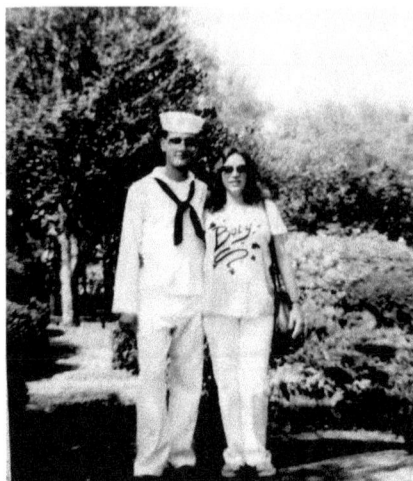

I was born in Portsmouth, Virginia's naval hospital on a Tuesday in August. My father served in the U.S. Navy as a quartermaster at that time. He had a skill for "rocking the boat," if you know what I mean. For him, the sea meant both connection and freedom. I was too young to understand what he meant by the paradox, let alone the secret of the sea. The world was my oyster, ripe with untasted possibilities. Everything seemed simple, yet for some reason, there was a yearning I couldn't explain.

Looking back, I understand what dad meant. The seas' ebbs and flows mirror the balance of freedom and restraint in our lives. Our experiences connect us to others, but sometimes these connections can feel like restraints. Like we're in handcuffs - and not the sexy kind.

The oceans' vastness symbolizes the freedom to explore - to find answers - to heal. But to successfully navigate the seas, we must embrace the ups and downs, and find balance between the storms that sometimes bind us and the freedom we seek. The sea is pure; it doesn't make excuses or hide what it is. And like the sea, we must lean into our authentic selves to guide us in finding the right balance for our lives.

We lived in Norfolk, nestled snugly at the mouth of the Chesapeake Bay. It was hot, and we didn't always have air conditioning. As a pint-sized rebel, I embraced my wild side, and clothes were more like optional accessories. Most days I ran around naked, getting into anything I could put my hands on. One warm day, my older brother and I thought we'd play Picasso in the kitchen, creating a masterpiece by liberating the fridge of its contents. Eggs were the crowd pleaser. I don't remember why, but I bet it had something to do with cooling off. Needless to say, Mom wasn't amused by our approach to temperature regulation. She always said I was a bona fide "nauti" girl.

And she was right! But let's keep that between us.

I am an explorer at heart, a true aquaholic in the nautical voyage of life. It is a very liberating space for me.

It's an adventure full of possibilities, risks, and pleasurable rewards. But naturally, we are bound to hit an iceberg sooner or later. Seemingly invisible at first glance, the real wreckage often lurks beneath the surface. I'm referring to the ongoing presence of trauma. That sneaky little t, or big T, can have lasting effects on our thoughts, emotions and responses if we fail to honor our struggles to create space for healing.

No one is coming to save us. We must learn to save ourselves.

Unfortunately, bad shit happens in good people's lives every day. But I believe life happens *for* us, not *to* us. In other words, yes, things happen, but we create the meaning! When stripped down, all life's experiences can reveal naked truths.

I am well aware you might not like or agree with this statement. If someone would have told me in the thick of my trauma that things are "happening for me," I might have throat-punched them. But now, I can accept the stories I'm about to share, and have chosen the purpose, the truth.

We are the captains of our ships. We have the steering wheel in our hands.

Feeling a bit adrift? No worries, it happens to the best of us. This journey's all about forward momentum.

None of us come equipped with a roadmap for every twist and turn, but as long as we're sailing ahead, fueled by our intentional choices we make and the habits we cultivate, we're on the right track.

I have firsthand experience with those moments that feel like the end of the world, staring down situations that made me feel physically ill. I remember times when just the thought of certain people or events made me sea sick for days, even weeks. Oh, I remember the feeling.

Have you ever been pulled under water into the depths of despair, making it hard to breathe? I'm making a brave assumption your answer is yes, because you're reading this book. So you understand, and I get it, I really do! And while I won't question your feelings, please know feelings aren't facts. Feelings are forms of energy in motion, and can be changed through our thoughts and words. Traumatic experiences pack a punch, no doubt. But I do not want to be a victim of my own life – I prefer to lead it. While I'm often unsure exactly why something is happening, I choose to reframe the energy as fuel to influence my future. This feels forward thinking, productive, and empowering!

Yeah, I know, easier said than done. But my intention for this book is to serve as a guide, helping us navigate our nausea in a way that awakens our sense of self-worth and resilience. Even in the worst moments of our life, there is something meant for us.

A lesson.

An experience.

A connection.

Life is always teaching us something. Pay attention.

We are all just students of life – which is happening *for* us.

Uncovering our naked truth from trauma can profoundly transform our lives when we embrace it as a gift. And we were all meant to share our gifts with the world.

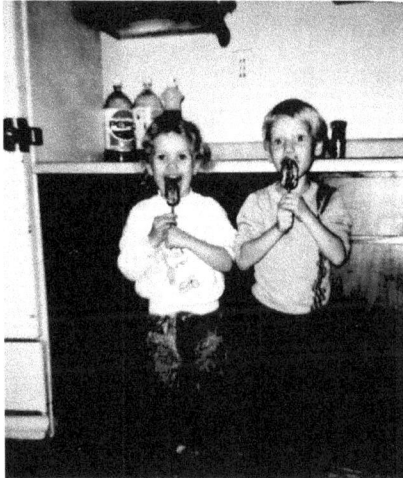

This is your invitation to throw off the bowlines, as we explore different dark places that hold the keys for growth, healing, and a life of fulfillment. I am no doctor or expert, but here's what I know to be true. So far I've survived 100% of my worst days. I am more than the terrible things that have happened. I admit, I'm not yet the person I have the capacity to be, but I'm damn proud of my commitment to the woman I'm becoming.

Whatever chapter of your life you're in, be in it - and know you're not alone.

CHAPTER 1

A Perfect Storm

"A smooth sea never made a skilled sailor."
—Franklin D. Roosevelt

In a culture consumed by tailored social media, filtered selfies, and self-righteous bullshit, can we all agree upon one thing? We are all bonded by the commonality of experiencing trauma in one way or another in our lives. Experiencing trauma does not mean we are destined for a life of hopelessness; it just means we should be aware of the patterns it can create if we refuse to acknowledge it.

All traumas can affect our self-worth, wellbeing, and connection to the world.

While some lives follow a smooth narrative, mine unfolded with numerous interruptions and pauses along the way. I've learned trauma has a way of unsettling the story. It rushes in, rattles everything, and then life goes on, leaving no map.

My family had a lot of dysfunction growing up; a perfect storm of pandemonium, the childhood edition. My whole life, I've had this unusual obsession with freedom and purpose. The idea was, life on my terms. However, I quickly learned that freedom did not exist in our home.

After my father completed his Navy term in Virginia, we all moved back to Wisconsin to be closer to family. My biological parents divorced when I was young. Back then, the court system decided on primary placement with Mom, and every other weekend with Dad. I had no strong feelings towards the arrangement. Dad remarried quickly, and he and my step-mother still live in the same house today. Mom too, found love again, an engagement ring, and shortly after the news of another baby boy to come.

Mother had always been hard-working, juggling multiple jobs to make ends meet - a strong Leo with a sense of loyalty and survival. She welcomed my independent spirit, was quite the Busch Light enthusiast, and a phenomenal cook with impeccable taste, except for in men at times.

Father had more masculine energy - the tough-love type; a minimalist, rigid, timely and tight with his money. He appeared well-balanced with a chip on both shoulders. Being a quartermaster in the Navy will do that to a man. Dad has the gift of gab, which I inherited. For him, everything had a place, and you better have known yours.

Despite their differences, my parents continually found common ground for the classic 'work hard, play hard' mentality. Education held a special place for both my parents, even though neither pursued college. For me, school was a haven - I put my heart and soul into studying, making friends for life, and excelling in both sports and academics. Most teachers and classmates were fond of my determination for future financial security, and relentless "disease to please" enthusiasm for life. Regardless of being different from my peers, nothing felt more important than fitting in. In general I was liked, except for the pungent smell of cigarette smoke that clung to my clothes.

The lunch ladies had this secret code of kindness, fully aware of our family's involvement in the free-meal program. They served more than just food, dishing out extra portions of empathy and understanding on the daily.

My relationship with my brothers wasn't the best, until we hit adulthood. Still, when the going got tough, we were there for each other. We were nomads, moving from place to place with Mom as her relationships crumbled one after another. Adult arguments became routine, especially when alcohol was in the mix. Verbal and physical abuse became all too familiar. We'd listen to Mom's tales of disappointment with every man in her life – cheating, misbehavior, and even shifts in sexuality – issues seeming to circle back to power and self-worth.

During my elementary school years, I was scared of my stepfather. His frustration with himself often transformed into anger directed towards my mom and us kids. My younger brother was diagnosed with ADHD when he was just five. Alongside his struggle to concentrate, he battled nocturnal enuresis (bedwetting). Our living situation at that time was in a bi-level duplex, with all the bedrooms upstairs. My brothers shared a room, and mine was situated next to theirs on the right.

Down the hallway with its specks of brown on the carpet lay the domain where Mom and our stepfather slept. Us kids tiptoed around, trying everything to avoid pissing him off. Success was rare. Mornings often felt like nightmares, filled with the echoes of either our stepfather's shouting, or him smacking my little brother for wetting the bed. I'd timidly peer out from my doorway, seeing my brother's face shoved into the urine-soaked blankets. It was a cruel display of dominance, adding to my brother's embarrassment and my stress induced anxiety.

Those guilt gripping memories still linger.

In moments of self-reflection, I question if I could've done more? Why didn't I ever speak up or tell anyone? Although there were rare moments when my bravery surged, I feared physical altercations and tears of my own.

It felt like us kids could never do anything right, even when we did nothing wrong.

As Mom's work schedule often kept her absent from the dinner table, our routine took on a disjointed cadence. Our stepfather's obsession with order and need for power kept us kids eating from triple-slotted, color-coded plastic plates - say that three times fast.

Sometimes I'd sneak into our pantry, stealing one of his mini powdered donuts from the bag just to spite him. Other times I would hide my pink plate, a small token of my "appreciation."

Often, his eyes were tinted red, like he hadn't slept in weeks. The smell of cologne, confusion, and skunk hung in the air - a mixture to mask his extracurriculars.

Despite my less-than-ideal upbringing, I never believed in its intentionality. Somehow, I sensed there would always be more storms to weather, and have come to trust that everything happens for us, not to us. **Life Happens For Us.**

This is an attitude of empowerment where we choose to create the life we want, rather than rejecting reality as it unfolds. Choices and decisions are power, projecting the definition of living in authenticity. As an act of self-worth, it means operating in alignment with who you are and what you want, intently participating in your own story. It ensures those around you embrace all that you are, including your trauma or those times when you feel triggered.

Trigger.

Ick.

What a loaded word.

Triggers embody strong negative emotional reactions in response to present experiences. But to keep within the theme, why don't we call them "anchors."

Sometimes anchors are obvious, but other times they are tricky and dredge up involuntary echoes of past trauma.

Anchors have us auditing ourselves.

Despite feeling immensely heavy, anchors are excellent indicators of internal healing that needs to be addressed. And admittedly, parts of me still feel weighed down at times.

No, this is not another spin on toxic positivity, the catch-all term often used for dismissing the genuine struggles people face in favor of an enforced sense of optimism. For someone navigating trauma, toxic positivity can feel invalidating. Or worse, one could feel disrespect and disregard for their experiences. This is not what I am suggesting though.

Breathe easy.

On the contrary, I'm saying we all have problems. We all have past wounds we are fighting through. We all carry trauma in some form.

And that's okay!

However, an essential responsibility remains; showing up and doing the deep personal work. I believe a crucial component of this work involves setting the intention to embrace a positive mindset and adopt an empowering attitude as we persist forward.

Time will march on, and eventually the inner turmoil quiets.

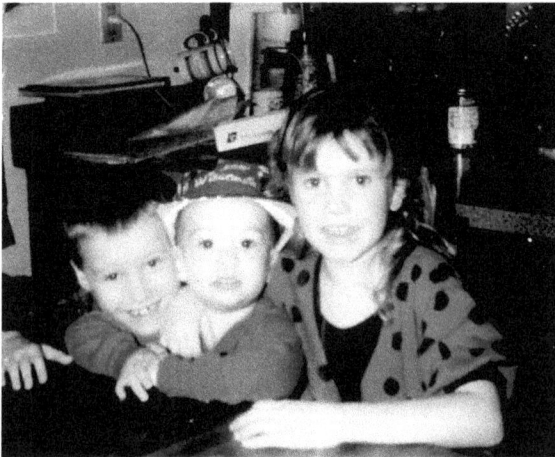

We come to embrace the notion that every twist and turn was essential in shaping us into who we are now. In this pursuit of belief, we inevitably experience growth while learning to heal at our own pace. It took me years to grasp this truth.

Life's experiences, the superb and the shitty, are gifts happening for us when we tune in and make the choice to recognize the benefit.

It is a perspective shift that pushes us to be active participants of our own lives. So, no matter what you experience, you can choose for it to make you grow in unbelievable ways.

CHAPTER 2

Invisible Anchors

"We don't have to wait until we are on our deathbed
to realize what a waste of our precious lives it is to
carry the belief that something is wrong with us."
—Tara Brach

There are many areas in everyday life that could use a makeover. At the top of my list is how trauma "recovery" is pursued.

In a world where recovering from trauma feels like a distant dream, many of us find ourselves trapped in a cycle of secret shame and unfulfilled expectations. It's society's hidden burden that presses heavily upon us. This weight, a subtle, invisible anchor designed to dictate our approach to both healing and the way we live. But I believe the key to healing is not found in the pursuit of recovery, but rather in the shedding of societal expectations. I believe the key to healing is embracing our unspoken realities, our "truthiest" truths – our naked truths.

However, I must confess, I don't know exactly what healing is supposed to look like. But that's also the beauty of it. Not having an expectation of what it's supposed to look like opens us up to the possibilities of what it can bring – healing on a deeper level.

My writing buddy April and I met for our weekly Zoom session as we always do. She began, "Alright Stephanie, what do you have for me this week?"

"I've been thinking about this for a long while... No one truly reaches complete recovery because the term itself is misleading," I explained to her, gesturing to the screen of the workshop we were participating in together. "Recovery suggests an endpoint that doesn't exist. Does that make sense?"

April pondered my words for a moment, her expression thoughtful. "So, you're saying that recovery isn't about reaching a destination, but rather about the journey itself?"

"Exactly," I affirmed with a nod. "It's about navigating the challenges, the daily ebbs and flows, to eventually find our own true north. I guess I can relate it to calibrating our internal compass. We just know it.
We feel it.
We stand in our authenticity.
And that's when we find our naked truth!"

"Interesting," she said as her eyes locked in a distant stare of concentration.

Nevertheless, I persisted, "I'm learning that trauma is a part of who we are. It will always be there, drifting below the surface. But when we honor its existence rather than chasing the idea of being completely healed, something amazing starts to shift within."

I began feeling at peace with all that has happened *for* me.

She chuckled, a hint of sarcasm on her face. "Kind of like steamboats, huh?"

Laughing so loud I almost spit my water out in response, remembering our inside joke from a previous writing session. "Oh gawd - steamboats. Back in the 1800's when Robert Fulton...," I stopped myself from going down that snoozefest again.

This book originally discussed way too much about steamboats and their history. I digress – and chuckle one more time. Writing is tough.

April and I ended our Zoom call with grace and gratitude.

* * * *

As you might have guessed, this book is not focusing on recovery. Instead, it emphasizes everyday healing; a process of continuously learning about ourselves. I provide ideas to empower us to coexist with our trauma and varied experiences – both positive and negative. Despite everything, my book underscores our ability to choose who we want to be, and how we build a relationship with ourselves first.

Embracing this mindset allows us all to deal and heal in the most advantageous ways.

My childhood environment became the breeding ground for a pervasive sense of lack that has influenced every aspect of my life.

Lack of awareness.
Lack of resources.
Lack of voice.

All lead to self-imposed limitations. That feeling and I, we have a long history together, rooted in prolonged exposure to powerlessness and the absence of accountability from those entrusted with my care. Like an invisible anchor, it strained my spirit, shaping my beliefs which supported the depletion of my self-worth account.

Even as an adult, the persistent sense of scarcity remains the heaviest anchor, dragging me down in unexpected ways. Memories flood back, snippets of conversations echoing in my mind, each one a reminder of the "*insufficiency mindset*" that has plagued me for years.

"Listen, money's really tight this month. We're just trying to cover the essentials, so we can't afford any extras right now."

"We're barely getting by as it is, so we've got to watch every penny."

"Hey, I get that you want stuff, but you've got to learn to appreciate what you've got. Some people don't even have a roof over their heads or enough food to eat."

"Sometimes you've got to do what you're asked without questioning it. It's just how things work around here."

"You know, there are starving people in other countries. Count yourself lucky."

"I know I sound harsh, but I'm just trying to make you understand. I brought you into this world, and I can take you out just as quick."

"Sometimes it's better to give up on something if it's causing you more trouble than it's worth."

Was I wrong for wanting more in life than food on my plate and a roof over my head? I always thought of myself as a grateful person, but let's be real, Salisbury steak and microwave fettuccine barely qualify as food. Can't I be both grateful and determined for something that ignites my inner Leo?

Why did I feel jealous of my friends going shopping and on vacation? Was it their material possessions or travels that sparked envy within me, or simply the sense of freedom and fulfillment they seemed to display.

Am I just greedy or full of desire? What's the difference? The distinction confused me as I struggled with the complexities of human nature. Was it wrong to yearn for more, to aspire to greater heights, or was it simply a reflection of my innate drive for growth and self-improvement?

I always understood desire as a natural longing for something perceived as lacking in one's life. I believe it arises from a genuine need or aspiration to improve one's circumstances, fulfill goals, or attain a higher level of satisfaction.

On the other hand, I believe greed is characterized by an insatiable craving for more, often at the expense of others or without regard for ethical considerations. It's often driven by a compulsive desire to accumulate wealth, possessions, or power beyond what is necessary or reasonable.

And yet both can still stem from a sense of scarcity and seeded belief that one is deserving of a fulfilling life – but according to who?

"Do I even deserve this life? Sometimes I wonder if I'm doing enough or if I'm just coasting through."

"Success... what does that even mean? And who gets to decide if I'm successful or not? It's like I'm constantly chasing this elusive idea without ever really knowing if I've caught it."

"I took some great photos on vacation, but I'm hesitant to post them. What if someone unfriends me again because they're jealous or annoyed by all the posts?"

"I don't get why we have to keep our new property purchase a secret. Shouldn't we be proud of what we've achieved? It feels strange to hide it."

"I'm really lucky to have found such a kind and supportive partner, but sometimes I wonder if I even deserve to be happy with him. It's like I'm waiting for something to go wrong."

Often I catch myself laughing out loud because my husband actually found me. You will hear this story soon. Funny how life happens for us.

So, can you relate? Do we share any common beliefs or desires? Perhaps deep down, we all yearn for something similar — ownership, confidence, reclaiming our power. None of our lives are perfect — mine certainly isn't. But amidst the imperfections lies the beauty, the potential for growth and transformation.

CHAPTER 3

Caught Between the Devil
and the Deep Blue Sea

"Time and Tide wait for no man."
—St. Marher, 1225

It's strange the things we remember from childhood.

As my four besties and I stood together, Ashley asked, "Steph, what's with the serious face? Aren't dances supposed to be, like, the highlight of our lives right now?"

"See that stuck-up priss over there flirting with my crush?" I blurted out, jealousy seeping from every pore.

"Who, her?" Kayla pointed to the skinny blonde laughing with my crush and his buddies. "She's like the queen bee of the bratty cheerleaders here at this school. Total attitude, that one," she added, flipping her brown curly hair with a dramatic flair.

"Yeah, well, obviously we (signaling to my girlfriends) don't go to this school and are only here for the winter soiree with those guys," I grumbled, jabbing my finger in the direction of our crushes. We were about as socially awkward as a bunch of sixth graders could be.

"Doesn't she know Adam is off-limits? Ugh, I need to do something," I insisted, feeling the need to defend my territory.

"You should totally give her a face full of nachos!" Kayla in our outcast group suggested with a mischievous glint in her eye. "Either her, or him," she pointed to one of Adam's friends.

Though I loved the idea, I couldn't do it. Not because I didn't want to, but I couldn't bear the thought of dancing with the devil if I got caught. I could already hear his raspy voice screaming at me in overreaction mode. My stepfather often needed a place to land his anger – my brothers and I were easy targets.

"What the hell, I'll do it," my rebel friend Kayla proclaimed, as she quickly walked over and shoved the cardboard container of yellow chips and gooey cheese in some dude's face.

Our instant OG group was solidified at that moment.

Kayla was the perfect addition to our girl gang. Cue the Set It Off soundtrack.

Friends can come and go in life. But sometimes, if we're lucky, they stick around for the long haul. To this day, us five remain the OG's.

Already on thin ice from the school incident, my stepfather was leery of our boy crazy band-of-misfits getting back together the following week to watch the guys' basketball team play. Our Banting Bobcats were up against the Hillcrest Huskies, where my aforementioned heartthrob just so happened to play. The wooden bleachers in the third row were practically shouting my name. And believe me, I was all set to scream my lungs out – for the game, of course! Excited and nervous to see Adam, I applied my game face in the mirror. The mirror winked back.

My stepfather's expectation was to be home at 9:00PM, which didn't bother me. I figured a few hours to drool over Adam's killer smile, lips that were practically made for snacking, and uncanny ability to chew gum like a pro was more than enough time. Gosh I liked him. But as "luck" would have it, the butt-numbing final quarter played long. Running short on time became my cardio. Just as I geared up for some flirtatious exchanges via note and sweaty hug, I had to rush home to the dry dock of missed opportunities.

The look of disapproval on my stepfather's face said it all, as I darted through the door. I underestimated the might of a few minutes, witnessing my power and freedom getting stripped away.

"You're late, Stephanie! Didn't I tell you not a minute past 9:00PM? Get upstairs to your room, now! You're grounded!"

Little did I know my seemingly innocuous 6-minute delay past curfew would trigger a tidal wave of consequences, including 6 long months of punishment for this 6th-grader.

There was no arguing with him – it would only make matters worse. I thought if I showed complacency, I might have a chance of getting ungrounded. However, learning to survive my stepfather kicked started my career in people pleasing and self-sabotage.

For the next half year, eleven-year-old Stephanie was on house arrest, courtesy of a man who wasn't exactly winning any "stepfather of the year" awards. It felt like an eternity behind bars, every thought and movement suppressed. "May I go to the bathroom," I would ask, my eyes fixed on a different scene just ten steps away from my personal cell block.

"Don't come out of your room until I tell you to," was a pretty common phrase yelled from the first level of the duplex.

The louder I became, the less I was heard.

Summer arrived – an almost intolerable season. While the neighborhood frolicked and kids laughed outside, my personal entertainment revolved around eavesdropping from the confines of my bedroom. I watched sparklers and fireworks burst in the sky from my window seat. The days of birthday parties, bike rides, and games like Ghost in the Graveyard felt like a distant memory in the museum of forgotten fun.

One evening, I stretched out on the soft carpet, face down, with my hands propping up my chin and palms nestled comfortably under my cheeks. I sank into the cozy embrace of the floor, recalling a specific memory from the previous summer.

My neighborhood BFF Ashley, who practically shared the same backyard, and I spent a lot of time together. Money was always tight, but whether building forts or selling dried flowers sprayed with perfume as "potpourri," we found a way to keep ourselves entertained on a budget.

Just beyond my squeaky patio door, I had a square slab of concrete in my backyard. It was perfect for the quintessential 90s plastic pool with flimsy sides that wobbled unless filled to the brim.

With no vacations on the horizon, Ashley and I decided to create our own adventure, filling the pool with water from the hose, and pretending it was our tropical paradise. Our imaginations took us to distant beaches with golden sand and turquoise water.

We spent hours crafting colorful pamphlets filled with exotic ideas. She and I talked about traveling to far-off places like Bora Bora, promising ourselves that one day we'd make it there. Regardless of being met with obstacles, neither she nor I allowed our dreams of wanting more, traveling, and changing the world to ever die.

* * * *

"This sucks. I miss my friends," thinking out loud. "I wonder what they are doing right now?"

Transitioning from the floor to my bed, I couldn't shake the feeling of loneliness and isolation. Every night I would lie there, staring at the ceiling, going over every detail and still wonder what I did wrong.

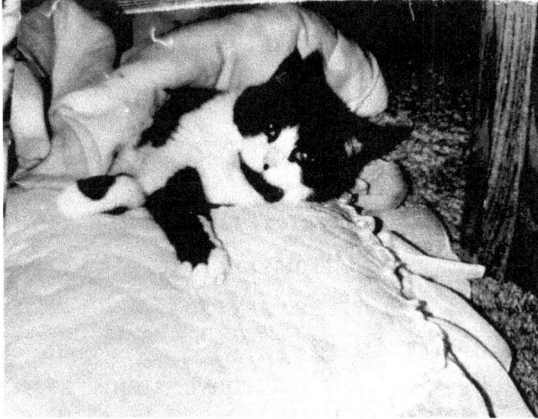

My hero among the confinement was none other than Oreo, my black-and-white feline friend and beacon of hope. We became an inseparable team, often stationed for hours just laying in bed or the doorway. Her soft purrs and warm nuzzles distracted me from the overwhelming sadness I felt. It was then that my profound love for cats truly blossomed, nurtured by their silent understanding and unwavering support. Oreo's presence became my refuge, a source of strength and solace during the most difficult of days.

I keep replaying memories of all the fun times with my friends, and it just makes me feel even more miserable. The silence in my room feels suffocating, and I wish I could escape this feeling of being trapped. Maybe tomorrow will be better...

Hope, smothered in "lack."

My stepfather had that kind of control over my life, over my mother's too.

CHAPTER 4

Deck Duel

"There is but a plank between a sailor and eternity."
—Thomas Gibbons

In Middle School, it only took two conversations, a few flashy smiles and one love note passed between classes to establish my relationship status with Horning's heartthrob, Dom. He, an eighth grade Adonis, was recently single after an unexpected breakup with the queen of the Mean Girls club herself.

Stacey, along with her posse of bullies, walked the hallways side-by-side in a wall formation, curly hair bouncing with each step. These girls thrived on making others feel small, using intimidation as their tool of choice. They were rough around the edges, yet self-assured with tongues as sharp as their fashion sense.

"Ugh, could you be any more awkward? It's like you're trying to embarrass yourself." "Nice outfit... if we were in kindergarten. Did your mom dress you this morning?" Sometimes there was even the occasional, "talk to the hand."

It felt like every remark was aimed at asserting dominance. I did my best to stay clear of them. I didn't care for drama, and certainly not her dissolved relationship status. It was hardly my problem, until suddenly it was.

For some reason, I fell for the bad boys – the edgy guys who were cool in a rebellious sort of way. The guys who didn't mind sneaking out at night. My new beau was all that, and a bag of chips. His confident swagger, yet mysterious vibe had me hooked and wanting to know more. In the arena of seventh grade romance, I was winning.

Shortly after everyone heard the news, other rumors began circulating. Stacey wanted to scare me - or teach me a lesson on "tough love." The typical drone of teenage chatter was interrupted by occasional snickers, whispers of "did you hear" or weird stares like I wouldn't notice. Oh, I noticed!

Most of my friends did their best to be cheerful and comforting. "Those girls are just jealous. Who cares what they say and think anyway? They are so dumb!"

Others clung to denial. "It's just a stupid rumor, Steph. What are they gonna do? They can't just leave school early to follow you home. Teachers are everywhere and someone will see."

"But would they see," I wondered?

My girlfriend Kari took a completely different approach to the situation. She had a plan - especially after stupid Stacey's friends went running their mouths in the locker room. "They better all watch their backs, including that skinny girl with the thick scrunchie." As if these dumb girls didn't see Kari and her cool new scrunchie standing behind them listening.

Outside the locker room, Kari approached me, "Don't worry girl. If they touch you, I'll tell my sister. Their ass will be grass!"

As the clock ticked towards the end of the day, the wait was torturous. So I grabbed my things, made up an excuse to leave class and went to the office. A tall receptionist holding a phone to her ear kindly stated, "go ahead and take a seat, I'll be right with you."

She's got to be kidding me, I thought to myself. *Wait? I didn't have time to wait.*

After what felt like an eternity, the last bell rang loudly, signaling the end of the school day. Jumping out of the seat, I ran as fast as I could from the office, out the front doors and all the way home.

Luckily, home was a few short blocks away.

Darting inside, I slammed the screen door, followed by the heavy main door, latching the chain lock. My backpack didn't make it past the entryway closet.

"Mom, are you home? Hello? Mom?" I shouted. There was silence.

About ten minutes passed, just enough time to settle down in the kitchen and grab a snack. The calm was rolling in. Maybe Stacey and company could talk the talk, but not walk the walk, I thought. That's good for me in this particular situation, as I took another bite out of my granola bar. Maybe the dim witts feel bad for me and will leave me alone?

Suddenly, a loud knock on the door interrupted my pity party. I ignored it - twice.

"Hello, anybody home. We know you're in there. Quit hiding from us" a raspy female voice from the other side of the door yelled.

Setting the wrapper on the table, I stood up, taking a deep breath. I wanted to show them I wasn't afraid. I wanted to show them they didn't have power over me. One slow step at a time, I walked over to my tiny foyer, nearly tripping over my damn backpack still sitting there.

"Let's just go in. She won't mind," another snickering voice childishly encouraged.

Opening the door, my eyes widened like a deer in headlights. The facade of courage shattered, as the girl gang and one guy burst inside. Their laughter and snarky remarks were overtaken by the clatter of my belongings and refrigerator being ransacked. My heart was pounding. I had no words.

"Alright, enough games," Stacey hissed. "You stole Dom from me, and now you'll pay." With a swift motion, she grabbed me hard, dragging me out of the house.

"No, stop it, blah blah," whatever pathetic pleas came screaming from my mouth. It didn't matter. No one was listening. One of the girls and the male accomplice decided to help themselves to my precious Oreo and Amaretto as well. "Leave my cats alone. Please. Take me but do not hurt them. Put them back!" Luckily, both feline friends were dropped in the grass before exiting the yard.

With a chorus of jeers and taunts, they paraded me down the street and around the corner, in perfect view of Ashley's house. It was the after-school hangout, always stocked with fun beverages and fruit snacks. Her blue duplex sat on the other side of the irrigation ditch from where I stood. I knew my OG's were all there. And the only thing standing in my way from Gushers and girl time were these pop tarts.

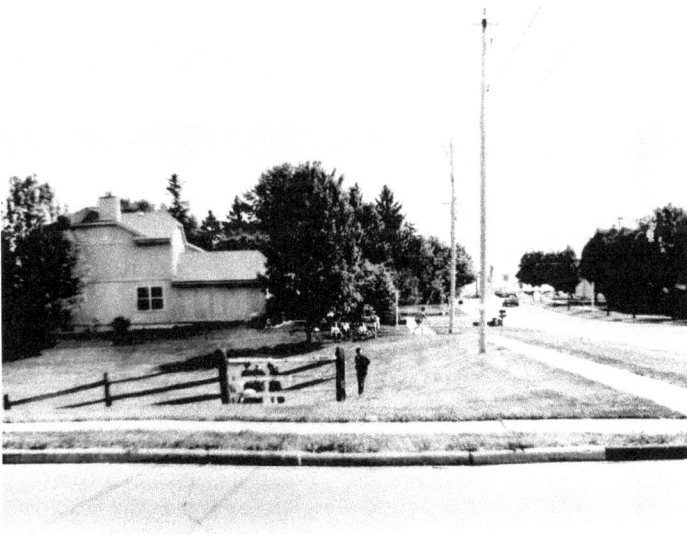

There in the open, on the stretch of sidewalk atop the ditch, my face met its very first fist. My wrists were tightly held behind my back like handcuffs, fingers ripping my hair to hold my head in place. Punches continued as tears streamed down my cheek.

Why aren't my friends helping me? Images raced through my mind as I believed they were watching me through the window. They have to see me. They have to see my scared 'I told you so' face.

With a surge of adrenaline-fueled strength, I broke free from the bullies and ran like hell. Stumbling my way through the patio door, I immediately felt relief seeing my cats back inside the house.

"Stephanie. What's wrong? What happened?" Mom questioned as the lines on her forehead deepened, showing the growing confusion that clouded her composed demeanor. "Why are you crying honey? Calm down and come here," she stated while walking down the staircase. "I can't understand you when you're crying like that." Mom's brows furrowed, her eyes darting around the room as if searching for answers in the air.

"Where the hell were you? I was beat up, Mom," I yelled.

"I was in the bathroom. What do you mean? I was here the whole time and heard nothing."

"Just forget it. You won't understand. Nobody does," complaining while running up the stairs to hide my adolescent embarrassment.

Bruised and ego broken, I vowed to break up with Dom.

The following morning I managed to wake up with my big girl panties on and decided to "show face" at school after all.

Fluorescent lights flickered overhead. Every step down the hallway felt like an eternal walk of shame. I caught pieces of words - lies, half-truths, and outright slander - typical middle school game of telephone. "Did you hear what happened? What a loser!" "Did she think she was something special?" "I can't believe she actually thought she had a chance with him?"

Although I publicly called off our adolescent relationship, Dom and I agreed to "keep things on the DL" for a while. He felt bad about everything, but didn't want it to prevent us from hanging out. Late night bike rides and secret sleepovers were apparently in my near future. So that helped.

Classmates noticed my abnormal quiet demeanor, the internal shame. There was no hiding my embarrassment from the microscope I was under. I allowed these girls to strip away my power and confidence. My flaws were exposed and I didn't know what to do. Every mundane task felt like a battle I was losing. My twelve-year-old self felt broken during a time I needed to build up my identity. I was just trying to survive the day.

In between classes, I noticed a few of my OG's by a locker. "What the heck. I thought you were my friends. I needed you, and you just watched?"

"What are you talking about, Steph?" Ashley questioned.

"Don't lie to me. I know you were all hanging out after school. I saw you watching through the window"

"Sorry girl, but we didn't see anything and don't know what you are talking about," Kari stated.

"So you're telling me you didn't see me when I was getting beat up?" Apparently I had convinced myself that my friends were watching and did nothing. The mind sure plays dirty tricks sometimes.

Before the day's end, Kari pulled me to the side. "Don't worry. I already told my sister what they did to you and how they threatened me too. She's pissed and will take care of it."

With a huge sigh of relief, "thanks. So what's she gonna do to help?"

"Well, after the spring dance when we all go to hangout, my sister and her friends are going to be there. Trust me, those bitches messed with the wrong girls. They don't even know what's coming!"

Secretly smirking while licking my wounds, I felt relieved that Stacey would get what she deserved.

Kari said, "you just wait!" So I just waited.

A couple of weeks passed. And after the dance as planned, a crowd of teenagers gathered at the popular spot, Burger King, for a little after-party fun. Some ordered food, while others chugged down soda outside. There were many faces in attendance, including stupid Stacey and her wannabees who didn't know what was about to hit them.

In the dimly lit parking lot, tensions and french fries boiled over as Kari's sister Tia arrived with her older friends dressed in dark clothing. Large, hoop earrings and high ponytails were ready to swing. They approached us first. "Stay behind us, sis" Tia said. "We've got this. No one messes with our crew."

Turning their attention to Stacey and her BFF Kloe, who we all also despised, their voices taunted, "Well, well, well, what do we have here?"

"You think you're pretty tough? Let's see how tough you really are" sneered a gang member.

With a sudden surge of aggression, insults turned into fists flying through the air. The chaotic symphony of shouting and shoving echoed off the concrete walls as the girl gangs clashed in a whirlwind of violence. Hands smacked Stacey's face, while locks and chains clawed at Kloe's defenseless body. Hair was ripped out – each side refusing to back down until the bitter end.

"I never wanted things to escalate this far," I renounced in the middle of the chaos, my guilt now weighing heavy on my conscience. My OG's and I stood frozen, unsure what to do. "I never wanted anyone to get that hurt. Maybe I should've handled things differently... I don't know. It's just a mess, and it's all my fault."

"We need to get out of here," Kari suggested just as a warning call came in.

"Everyone run! Berries and cherries – time to go," a harsh voice shouted in the distance. I saw the police cars fast approaching, and frantically ran in the opposite direction. All bystanders scattered like farts in the wind.

Days following, under the shade of the slide at the local park, our OG crew gathered." I... I can't believe it went down like that," I murmured, my voice barely above a whisper, my hands fidgeting nervously. "I mean, part of me feels relieved, you know? Like, finally getting some payback after all she's done. But seeing her end up in the hospital... It's just too much."

"Yeah," Kayla nodded solemnly. "I heard she's in critical condition."

"Do you think we'll get caught?"

"Well, Tia was already cuffed and taken to juvie that night. Someone ratted her out."

Though regret has faded with time (and an apology within the past decade), the memory of that night still lingers as a reminder of the fragility of life and the depths of our own darkness.

As we stood there in the silence of our own guilt, we exchanged concerned glances that held collective remorse.

"We almost killed her."

CHAPTER 5

Siren's Song

"While lying bare, open, and choiceless as a beach,
the sea will still come bearing gifts"
—adapted from Anne Morrow Lindbergh

It's much easier to talk about the weather, sports, or the latest gossip than it is to share our unfiltered experiences with trauma. Life isn't always wrapped in a pretty bow, but it still remains a precious gift. And, the more we hide from these truths, the more time we waste idle in life's shadows.

I debated sharing this next story with you. It's one of the darkest moments of my life (anchor warning)...

When wool socks and shovels are finally put away for the season, us vitamin D-deprived Wisconsinites are ready for great fun in the sun. As school let out, it meant manicured lawns, concerts, barbeque and boating season was upon us. You could smell the anticipation emanating from around the state.

No longer delegated to the bottom of the high school food chain, the "I want to experience it all" mentality gripped me as I eagerly awaited the end of the month, when the world's largest music festival would unfold in the bustling city of Milwaukee. Set against the scenic backdrop of the lakefront, Summerfest promised a smorgasbord of shows, local food, refreshing drinks, and shopping opportunities galore. Thousands of people gather to attend this annual iconic event.

"Finally, it's my turn," I thought. "Fourteen and feeling like I'm practically an adult already." I was so excited, with the song "Summer

Girls" by LFO playing on repeat in my head. But although I felt like an adult, the reality was I still had to rely on others for transportation.

"Hey Steph, my friend and I were thinking of heading down to Summerfest. Wanna come along?" asked Kevin, a familiar face who was of legal drinking age.

"That sounds awesome, thanks!" I replied. "Let me chat with Krista first."

Youthful and trusting, I spoke with my friend. "Don't worry! I obviously know him and heard about his buddy. Just tell your mom you're sleeping over and let's go have some fun."

We happily agreed to go have some fun. At our age, we tend to trust people close to us and trust their friends will treat us the same way as they do.

When Kevin and his buddy JP showed up, I couldn't help but notice JP's easy smile and confidence. Admittedly, I was attracted to him. His sleek yellow muscle car, a flexing symbol of his personality, drew me in fast. I was excited for the adventure to unfold.

Just as I hopped into the back seat, Kevin offered me my first cold Zima. "Here, you should totally try this!"

I grinned, feeling my vibrant spirit come alive. "Sure, why not?" I replied, eager to impress and experience something new.

"I haven't really had alcohol before," I disclosed.

"It's like clear soda, really refreshing," he reassured me.

Curious and a bit giddy with anticipation, I took a sip, finding it surprisingly enjoyable. "Hmm, not bad," I said, feeling the bubbles tickle my tongue. "Krista and I will take a few back here."

The evening was full of laughter and my favorite tunes. Bouncing around from stage to stage, we danced our asses off while continuing our under-age drinking. Garbage cans were overflowing. People-watching was on point. Vendors and dated picnic tables lined the lakeshore. When the wind blew just right, the tempting smell of candied nuts was enough to sweep anyone off their feet.

Eventually the sensory overload would calm down, as the people made their way to the exit. The four of us piled back into the car. Decision making skills were out the window, and the night would end much differently than it began.

My guard was down.

Leaving Summerfest, we headed to JP's apartment. Soon upon entry, JP and Kevin began bickering. I couldn't help but feel annoyed at the buzzkill. Seeking solace from the tension, I quietly slipped into JP's bedroom.

To my surprise, he followed me right in. His presence sent a message. Before I knew it, we were sitting on the bed, our lips kissing in the dark. I couldn't help but feel a rush of adrenaline. At my naive age, a tipsy makeout session like this was something worth bragging about.

I remember feeling tired and ready to pass out, when he removed his sweaty gray shirt. Laying next to me, we continued fooling around. He began acting aggressive and took his pants off, wanting me to join him below deck.

Everything felt wrong.

His muscular, over six-feet tall body rolled onto me. Pushing his hips back, he thrust forward. "No, eh, no, I don't like this, no, stop," I repeatedly urged, trying to shove him away.

"No, stop, I'm not comfortable, no," I pleaded while squirming. As if my intense non-verbal's weren't enough, my heart was pounding so intensely, I thought it was going to jump out and punch him.

Why won't he stop? What the hell doesn't he understand? The question lingering on my lips, colored with a hint of self-doubt. Things continued for what felt like an eternity, but probably a few minutes. My demands were eventually silenced with misty eyes.

There I was, lying helpless in his white bedding, painted in red. He – still holding the power.

Full of shame, resentment, and lord knows what else, I passed out for an unknown time.

My friend Krista had apparently also dozed off in the living room. Feeling both embarrassed and indebted, I didn't know how to respond to her knock on the bedroom door. "Steph, are you awake in there? I think we should go. We need to get back."

Alarmed, I initiated auto-cleanup mode as fast as possible. Krista was right. It was morning and we needed to get home, but how I thought to myself?

"Go ahead, I'll take care of it," JP stated.

Yea right. What was he thinking? Like I'd just forget. Did he want to touch me again? So many voices running through my head. It would be a cold day in hell when I let that happen.

Deliberately ignoring his gesture, I walked to the bathroom where my friend greeted me as I entered. "Hey, so how are we getting home?" she asked. "We should probably call your mom – and make up something."

Luckily, her parents thought she was sleeping over at my house. What the hell am I going to tell my mom, I wondered.

We slipped out the front entryway of the old brick covered apartment. Our bloodshot eyes were met by the sun. And after a deep breath, I mustered the courage to call my mother to pick us up. Making up some story, I lied about what we did, where we slept, everything. This was not a proud daughter moment.

No one could find out about that night's events, not even my good friend Krista. What had started as a quest for fun, unexpectedly turned into the path less traveled.

Arriving home, my emotions were messy.

Somberness. Confusion.

Tears I have kept hidden for so many years.

As my friend left, I sank onto my bed, feeling a deep sense of disbelief washing over me. How could he fail to comprehend that my repeated pleas of "no," "stop," and "I don't want to" were clear indications that I did not welcome his advances?

The weight of misunderstanding and betrayal was heavy upon me. I was lost in a sea of uncertainty and hurt.

He should have come with a warning.

His scent lingered on my skin, polluted with the truth.

Rape. There, I said it.

What a gross word. You don't forget something like that though.

It was the first time I experienced sex. Unfortunately, it lacked all the things that are supposed to make it fun; mutual consent, connection, vulnerability and respect. Learning about sex from rape is like trying to learn about the ocean from a burnt sea breeze candle.

It's fake.

It's ugly.

It's jaded – exposing its use. I feared fake sex would ruin real sex for me forever.

When I got home, I took two showers to scrub JP from my body, but I couldn't wash the experience from my life.

Then, I entered into a downward spiral, a fun laced with problems era within just a few short months. Despite my best efforts, I found myself unable to practice the mindfulness and discipline needed to control my drinking and recognize when I'd had enough.

A flood of emotions and phases followed, particularly a brutal sophomore year. Things went downhill at an alarming rate. Waves of outrage and reckless partying swept over me. At first, I couldn't understand where it was coming from – rather I didn't want to. Rumors began to swirl about my newfound habits and sexual escapades. Although I had been intimate with others since the traumatic experience, none of them held any real significance for me. My attention-seeking behavior was a direct reflection of the powerlessness I felt in the aftermath.

The news reached my father, likely through the grapevine of my older brother. During a painful phone conversation, he lashed out at me with derogatory remarks and accusations about my character. That was the last time my father and I spoke for over a year.

My neighbor, and basketball coach that year, was the only person I felt not judging me. The only person who seemed to offer understanding was him. Coach noticed the subtle shifts in my social, emotional, and physical demeanor, probing gently with questions that cut deeper than I was ready to confront. He saw through me like an open book, but not the kind I was prepared for anyone to read.

Slinking into the shadows, I couldn't escape the tears that flowed freely during sports practice. Weekends became a minefield of uncomfortable situations I'd rather have avoided. As if that wasn't enough, I ended up benched for a whopping five basketball games – clearly, my aggressive spirit wasn't appreciated.

This was also the year women's pole-vaulting came into the high schools. Naturally, who better than a sassy, manic teenager like me to take on the challenge of a new risky field event?

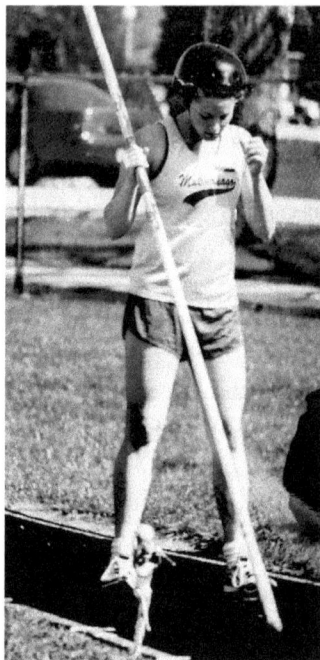

One day during track practice, the pole-vault coach called me over to the vault area. He handed me a pole and said, "Just go for it." Without hesitation, I took the eleven foot pole from him and nodded. Determined to give it a shot, I visualized propelling myself upward – over my issues. So with zero clue what I was doing, I sprinted down the runway, planted the pole in the box, and launched myself into the air.

As I soared, I could hear the coach cheering me on from the sidelines, yelling something about having the courage to try something new. Damn it felt good!

Pole-vaulting quickly became my obsession. It was the perfect distraction from everything else going on in my life, and eventually, it became exactly what I needed.

CHAPTER 6

Red Treasure Chest

"Whiskey is for drinking. Water is for fighting"
—Mark Twain

The sky was clear as I drove home from school. My muscles ached from track practice, and my mind was consumed with thoughts of homework and my part-time job. I was a teenager and going to be the first in my family to go to college; every penny I earned was a step closer to that dream. As I approached the duplex where we recently moved (again) into, I allowed myself a moment of pride.

Walking into the house, I was greeted by the familiar scent of home – baking oil and laundry detergent. Mom was in the kitchen, listening to country music softly – an evening when she was not at work. Her weary eyes lit up when she saw me, a brief respite from her constant worries. I greeted her with a warm hello before heading upstairs to my room. Exhausted from the day, but it didn't matter. I still had homework to finish.

School.

Practice.

Work.

Homework.

Rinse and repeat.

This was life for the time being. At least I recently switched jobs for an extra buck and a half an hour. Just as I opened my math book, I became distracted with the thought of money. I wonder how much I have saved up so far? Eager to count, I jumped off the bed to grab my little red treasure chest made of metal. Then, my stomach dropped as I spotted it in the corner – the busted remains of my treasure chest on the carpet floor. My savings – nearly $2,000 in cash – had been wiped clean, stolen right out from under me.

My heart, a melting pot of anger and angst. I knew with every ounce of my being who had done it. My little brother was only 14 but had already found trouble more times than I could count. Still, I wanted to give him the benefit of the doubt as I always found myself doing. I wanted to believe in him. I wanted this to be a simple misunderstanding.

Clenching my fists, trying to steady my breath, a wave of panic came crashing in. The walls of my room seemed to engulf me, the space that was my safe haven now felt suffocating.

"Moooooommmmm!" screaming from the top of my lungs as tears came flooding out. She couldn't hear me, and I had no idea where anybody else was, nor did I care.

Crawling back into bed, I couldn't fathom the situation at hand.

* * * *

A few weeks later, the second wave of anger hit me when I woke up to find my car "missing."

At first glance out the window, I was unable to spot my Eagle Talon shimmering in the sun. Rushing outside, it was parked differently than I had left it, and now covered in mud with corn husks in the wheel wells.

Red with rage and disbelief, I realized that the little shit of a brother had taken it for a joyride. After confronting him, he naturally denied everything - eyes wide with fake innocence.

"I know it was you! Why would you do this to me?" I demanded, my voice shaking with anger. I could feel my blood pressure rising, my vision blurring at the edges with fury.

"I didn't do anything, Stephanie! You're always blaming me for stuff I didn't do!" he retorted, his defiance infuriating me even more. His words were like knives, each one twisting deeper into my gut.

"Blaming you? You think this is about blame? Look at my freaking car! Do you think it drove itself through the cornfields?" My voice cracked, the hurt and frustration pouring out.

My little brother crossed his arms, his face a mask of annoyance. "Maybe if you weren't always so busy with your perfect little life, you'd see that I have problems too! But no, it's always about you and your stupid shit!"

I was stunned into silence, the weight of his words pressing down on me. My goals, my hard-earned money, my car – all seemed trivial in that moment compared to the rift growing between us.

Shortly after the car incident, the breaking point came knocking one evening post work. Exhausted and hungry, I opened the refrigerator to indulge in the one luxury I allowed myself – expensive red raspberries. But they were gone. Every single one. I saw red, not from the raspberries but from the rage returning inside me. I knew, once again, it was my little brother. I could feel it in my bones.

I yelled his name, storming through the house. The creaky floor beneath my feet felt like a ticking time bomb, each step bringing me closer to an inevitable explosion. "Where are you, you little piece of shit?"

"Stephanie, quit your swearing," Mom yelled in the background.

He was in the living room, sprawled on the couch amidst a pile of empty snack wrappers. He looked up at me with a smirk that only fueled my anger.

"What do you want now?" he asked lazily, his tone dripping with disdain.

I lost control. "What do I want? I want my freaking money back! I want my car cleaned! And I want my goddamn raspberries!" I screamed, grabbing a pot from the kitchen. "Do you have any idea how hard I work for this? Do you even care?"

His smirk disappeared, replaced by fear as I advanced on him. "Stephanie, calm down! It's just raspberries!"

"Just raspberries?" I screamed, swinging the pot. "It's everything! It's my money you stole, my car you stole, my future! You take everything, and disrespect me! I'm done!"

My brother raised his hands defensively, backing away. "You don't understand! It's not a big deal, dang! I didn't know they were your raspberries. You always think you're better than everyone!"

His words repeated in my mind, a perfect blend of deflection and "poor me excuses."

But underneath my rage, something else stirred – something I didn't want to face. We had both been hurt, both carried the weight of our past, but while I tried to rise above it, he was letting it fester. My anger wasn't just about the raspberries, the car or the cash; it was the frustration of watching him succumb to the similar trauma that I was desperately trying to escape.

"Maybe if you actually tried to do something with your life instead of ruining mine, things would be different!" I shouted back, blood boiling as I whacked his arm with the pot.

"I hate you," I shouted while hitting him again... and again.

But it wasn't just him I hated at that moment. It was the feeling of powerlessness, the echoes of our shared childhood trauma rumbling between us. We were both products of storms, but while I had fought to rise above the wreckage, he seemed determined to sink deeper into it, dragging me down with him.

I realized then that the cycle of pain we were trapped in wasn't just his doing or mine – it was a consequence of our past.

The fight was ugly.

My mother's frantic call to the police landed me in loads of trouble. By the time the officers arrived, I was exhausted, both physically and emotionally. They handcuffed me and charged me with disorderly conduct and battery. The look on my mother's face was one of utter devastation.

A part of me felt a deep, distracting pain from the realization that my own brother had intentionally betrayed me, his big sister... again.

Another part of me felt guilty, knowing that some of the same trauma that shaped me into someone who fought to survive had left him feeling like he had no choice but to keep playing the victim.

The trauma of that day has stayed with me, weighing me down like an anchor even after all these years. The hurt, anger, and betrayal I felt toward my brother never really faded. Despite the saying that "blood is thicker than water," I've struggled to get onboard with that idea.

I've come to realize that family isn't just about blood; it's about the people who show up for us with unconditional love and unwavering support. Sometimes, the ones who lift us up aren't the ones we started this journey with, but those who throw us a lifeline in the water when we need it most.

Water, the very essence of life, can heal us, connect us, and sustain us. But it can also drown us if we're not careful. It's a force of nature, just like the relationships we choose to nurture or let go. We get to decide who we let into our lives, who we swim alongside, and who we leave behind.

Water is life. Water is death.

The choices we make determine whether we sink or swim.

CHAPTER 7

Sinking Ship

"The sea is an incarnation of emotion incarnate. It loves, hates, and weeps" —Yvette Depaepe

Every relationship story holds clear truths and dirty lies, making them impossible to capture accurately from a single perspective. I had a love affair with self sabotage, especially when it came to romantic relationships.

I tried changing who I was, seeking love outside myself. This tactic will never work – in life or relationships.

Well over a decade ago, when my boyfriend at the time had been repeatedly unfaithful, I still wasn't sure if I'd leave him.

I had just completed my undergrad, and had a shiny new bachelor's degree in hand. Upon returning to my home area, I was greeted by its small-town charm of scenic lakes and live music. Anticipation buzzed inside me as I looked forward to a season filled with events and reunions with friends.

One warm evening as the rock band played its last song, a large, alcohol impaired crowd began clearing out from the festival tent. My eyes widened and mouth dropped, captivated by the presence of a dark featured man, standing no more than fifteen steps away.

"Hey, gorgeous," he shouted with his radiant smile and magnetic personality. The surprise on my face said it all. He remembered me from last year!? Is he single now? Wish I could say the same, I thought to myself, still mixed up with my college boyfriend in our sinking "it's complicated" status-ship.

You see, Adam and I had been "together" for three years. He was a total romantic and a killer DJ, which sounds perfect – until the late nights and partying led to drinking, flirting, and, eventually, cheating. Breaking up should've been simple, but when you're practically part of each other's families, walking away felt more like trying to end your favorite song that had been playing on repeat for so long.

"Hey handsome! I wasn't sure I'd run into you here." My subtlety was overridden by my blushing face.

"Well, I'm glad you did. How have you been?" he asked as we hugged.

"Seeing as I just graduated and moved back, I'm fantastic. You?"

"I'm good. Sounds like we have a lot of catching up to do," he insisted.

Mister Charismatic and I didn't leave before exchanging phone numbers. We technically met through mutual friends the summer prior – when social media was in its infancy stages and we both were romantically involved with other people.

I was not about to wait another year to see him. Hell, I wasn't going to wait an extra day to reach out either.

The next morning my phone call to Jason was met with an invitation to come over and go boating with his friends. I dove headfirst at the opportunity to get to know him better, and show off my wakeboarding skills of course.

With a shared zest for life, we seamlessly blended into the same social circles, making every moment spent together charged with excitement.

As summer unraveled, so did our love story, just in time for the long overdue breakup with my college boyfriend. Infectious laughter, intense passion, and a wild sense for adventure seemed to speed up time as Jason and I became inseparable. Goal-focused conversations, and fast sportbike excursions provided a sense of renewed vitality in me. It wasn't long before that I secured my own motorcycle license, equipped with vibrating 1125 CC's between my legs.

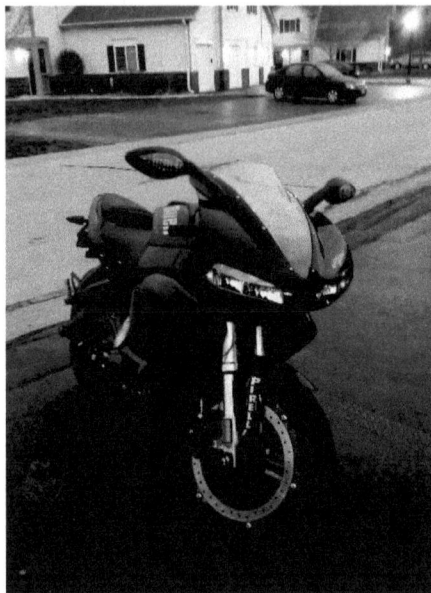

Eventually, I moved in with Jason and we settled into his house, mapping out our future together. We sat on the couch, surrounded by color swatches, watching an episode of The Walking Dead, and I couldn't help but to think, *I'm in trouble now*. I sure was falling hard!

After my serious college relationship ended, I was terrified to open up again. Jason was the first person I trusted enough to share my heart – and a home – with. We painted the walls with promise, bought new furniture to match, and every decision felt like another yellow brick laid on the road to our perfect future.

But even as we picked out shades of blue-gray and beige, there were shadows lurking in the corners. Moments when I would catch him texting someone, his phone angled just out of my view. Or how he'd casually mention running into his ex and then brush it off like it was nothing. I ignored it at first, convinced that everything was going so well, it couldn't possibly be a problem.

One evening, Jason and I went countertop shopping. "What do you think about this color and pattern?" he asked, his voice filled with optimistic confusion. I smiled, choosing the blue fleck granite without realizing that below the surface, cracks were starting to form.

As time passed, the canvas of our future began to reveal unexpected shades of gray – not the fifty kind.

Tension crept in quietly. The bedroom, once filled with sultry love and laughter, now felt heavy with words unspoken.

It all boiled over one night after we returned from the bar. I stood by the bed, arms crossed, staring at him, my heart aching from betrayal.

"Why do you keep doing this to me?" I demanded, my voice trembling. "You know how much it hurts me when you continue associating with those girls, especially your ex's when they talk shit about me. You flirt with them right in front of me, and you know they're still in love with you!"

He shifted uncomfortably, avoiding my gaze as guilt flashed across his face. "I don't know what you're talking about, we're just friends," he mumbled, his words failing to mask the truth. "Quit being so crazy."

"You're the crazy one, lying to me and thinking you can get away with it!" I exclaimed, my frustration spilling over. "I've seen the messages; I've heard the rumors. You're cheating on me, and completely disrespecting our relationship every time you do it."

Jason sighed heavily, clearly frustrated. "You're just insecure," he insisted. "You're not going to control who I'm friends with and who I'm not. You're crazy – always blowing everything out of proportion," his tone defensive – lips dripping honey Jack.

Dispensing tears, I shook my head in disbelief. "I can't do this anymore," my choked up voice barely above a whisper. "I deserve better than this. I deserve someone who respects me, who values our relationship and loves me."

Jason turned his back on me, clearly indifferent. "Oh, here we go again, Stephanie's crying. Just stop, please."

"Don't walk away from me when I'm talking to you. It's so fucking rude," I pleaded, my voice thick with desperation. "Wait, I'm sorry. I'll change, I promise. I'll do whatever it takes to make things right." I might as well be wearing a 'doormat' sticker on my forehead.

I knew this argument was just the beginning of the end.

Jason had this way of me believing I couldn't do better – that I was crazy – and fighting was always my fault. There I went, questioning my own worth, again.

Deep down, my gut knew the truth.

Dirty little lies.

Empty promises.

Our relationship played like a broken record, stuck in repetitive arguments, brutal break-ups and magical make-ups. We even thought a trip to Sin City would reignite the spark between us.

"Steph, even though we argue a lot, I'm in love with you," Jason declared, dropping to both knees and slipping a ring onto my finger. Wrapping my arms around his muscular frame, I held him close as I gazed out the large hotel window. I couldn't help but wonder if this was the moment everything would change for us.

"Oh gosh, yes, I want that," I giggled, just before my warm breath whispered, "I love you so much!" There was obviously more I wanted to say, but held back so as to not ruin the moment – or our getaway. However, the voice inside my head continued to grow louder. Can I trust him again? A promise ring – if he planned to stay and love me forever, why not actually propose?

I wanted this so badly I continued sweeping the red flags under the rug. I was the rug.

Toxicity continued creeping into our relationship for years, casting shadows of doubt as other women and insecurity still lingered in the background. Our once steamy bond seemed to be evaporating as we found ourselves at a crossroads. He clearly didn't look both ways before jumping in bed with someone else again.

Turns out, he wasn't in love with me the way I thought.

Jason's job had him traveling a lot, days – sometimes weeks on end. Then one night while out of town, the phone call came in.

"Hey hun – *silence* – what's wrong?"

Jason said something along the lines of, "Steph, this clearly isn't working. I don't want this relationship anymore. I'm ending this for good."

"Wait, what? Are you serious – stop saying that? There's somebody else you met isn't there? How can you do this when you said forever?" emphasizing our past promises. "I love you!"

As I uttered those three words – words that held so much weight for me – I waited with baited breath for his response. "Yup, love you too," came his hesitant reply. His words lacked the sincerity I had hoped for, and I knew they were a means to an end.

"Why are you doing this? We can work through things and figure it out," I pleaded!

"Steph, I understand that this is difficult, but what did you expect? Let's be realistic here. We both know that we're not compatible, and it's clear that our relationship isn't working. I think it's best if you find somewhere else to live so we can both move on with our lives. Take your time to find a new place; there's no need to rush into anything."

The phone call wasn't the only thing ending in that moment.

Why doesn't he love me? How can I ache in places I didn't know I had? What do I do now?

I saw this coming, didn't I? So why does it still sting? I should have called it quits with him years ago. I shouldn't have snooped through his stuff. I shouldn't have listened to his empty promises...

I was shoulding all over myself.

My best friend Liz repeatedly counseled me until blue in the face. "I understand feeling shitty, scared, and insignificant as humanly possible. You will find someone else Steph. Your heart loves, but think about all the crappy things he's done. You two are oil and water."

"How in the hell could I believe we were happy for so many years," questioning my own judgment.

It didn't matter how much I screamed or worked out, or how many shots I drank or conversations with friends took place. Every night I would lay in bed, stare at the ceiling, go over every detail and still wonder what I did wrong.

One month later and ten pounds lighter, I moved into an apartment just outside Milwaukee, nestled within a neighborhood characterized by lower socio-economic status and vibrant diversity. Concerns echoed from my friends and family, including my mother, who worried about my safety and well-being in such an environment. Despite their apprehensions, I was drawn to the opportunity presented by my buddy's parents, who owned a dental office in the area. They generously offered me the chance to reside upstairs for a mere three-hundred dollars per month.

It was a steal!

As I settled into my new living situation, I found comfort in decorating my spacious abode with all my previous belongings, including my two beloved furry companions, Malibu and Bailey.

Here, I continued my Masters degree program. After losing my identity in a five year relationship, it was time to refocus on myself and search for new meaning. Connecting with old friends, working multiple jobs and finishing school was the perfect distraction.

After sleeping over at my girlfriend Jaci's house, I returned to my apartment early the next morning from a restless night out. As my seafoam green Volkswagen, hot pink high heels and I pulled into my driveway, fatigue was setting in, mirroring the emotional exhaustion I still felt.

"Hey, I have to let you go. Something is not right and Bailey is outside," cautiously ending my phone call with my stepmother and turning off the car. Approaching the first of two entryway doors up to my apartment, I grabbed my cat from the lawn while reeling in my elevating pulse.

Why is the main door cracked open, I thought to myself? Crap, did I forget to close it on my way out? Kicking it shut, I turned the corner and immediately noticed my other cat Malibu. I then peered up the flight of stairs to my actual apartment door. Each step became faster than the next, until I was looking directly into my kitchen through a large hole.

Dropping Bailey and sinking to my hands and knees, my fingers traced the cool surface of the laminate floor. Feeling violated throughout my entire body, I thought I was going to puke. Pictures that once hung on the wall were on the floor. The broken glass was sharp against my skin, each piece a reminder of my shattered feelings.

The only thing I knew how to do when feeling pissed, powerless and triggered – I ugly cried!

Items were rummaged and thrown everywhere. My tears bounced off the empty walls, but there was nothing I could do. The damn anchors – powerlessness and violation – were rearing their faces again.

Running from the kitchen, down the hall to my living room, I found my wrap-around couch intact, but all my electronics were missing.

"No, this isn't happening. Please God, please," I begged to the big man above - or whoever was listening.

Still fearful, still crying, but now crawling down the hall back to my office space, the worst was yet to come.

"Oh God, no. Wake up Stephanie. This is just a nightmare," pleading and slapping myself before letting out a monstrous sobbing scream. In that moment, empty was something both the room and I had in common.

My laptop, backup drives, flash drives, everything had vanished! By everything, I even mean my ninety page master's thesis due in under two months for graduation. My chest tightened as the nauseating feeling overtook my body. Curled up in the fetal position, I convulsed with the thought. What did I do wrong this time? Was I calling too much attention to myself in this neighborhood? Should I have listened to my family regarding their concerns about moving to this side of town where crime was high?

Just as I began feeling proud of my accomplishments and the direction I was heading, swines swooped in and snatched it all away from me.

Inching my way to my bedroom, jewelry and hangers pierced the carpet. The bedding was in disarray, like the aftermath of newlyweds on their honeymoon night. Shit, they even took my laundry basket full of dirty clothes. Shaking in desperation, I reached for my phone and dialed... No matter how much time has passed, the only person I wanted most at that moment was Jason.

"Hello, Steph? Wha, what's wrong? Slow down – I can barely understand you. Where are you at? I'll be right there!" Without hesitation, he offered to be by my side.

About twenty minutes later, still frantic on the floor, my knight in shining armor rushed through the door. I'm not sure what looked worse, my apartment or my wet slobbery face.

Hugging each other amidst all the turmoil, we felt the spark of the love that had brought us together in the first place. We held onto that moment like a lifeline, hoping it would guide us through yet another storm.

The weeks after the break-in left me feeling disgusted and terrified. I spent countless evenings curled up in bed, staring at the ceiling, holding my breath as I replayed every detail in my mind. The nights were the hardest, with every sound resembling doors creaking open. Gunshots and the wail of sirens echoing in the air didn't help matters either. One particularly unsettling recollection was being startled awake by a late-night call.

"Hello, who is this?" I demanded, now up, pacing back and forth, and heart racing with anxiety. In the background, I could hear squirting noises, adding to my unease. Confusion grew as the muffled voice of a strange man began moaning and panting, sending shivers down my spine.

"I'm smelling your underwear and it makes me so horny," the disturbing voice claimed.

My palms began sweating, "is this some sick joke? Who is this?," tone trembling with fear and disgust.

"These are your pink and black panties. I know because I took them. I've been watching you," the deep voice emphasized.

Abruptly hanging up the phone, the anticipation of starting a new lease near my father's house couldn't come fast enough.

After picking up the pieces once again, the weight of disappointment and false expectations pressed heavily upon me. Despite our considerable attempts to mend our relationship, Jason and I found ourselves grasping at makeshift solutions – band aids, adhesive, and hope – to hold us together.

After nine more months of struggling and one detailed note of a sexcapade found in his suitcase, we reached the inevitable end of our chapter and parted ways – for real this time.

CHAPTER 8

Plenty of Fish

"On a day when the wind is perfect, the sail just needs to open and the world is full of beauty." —Rumi

Curled up on our cozy beige couch, draped in blankets, my roommate B and I indulge in our favorite pastime - watching reality TV in our pajamas. Her superpower was making wine disappear. So, with glasses of red vino in hand, we settle in for a night of laughter and drama. My roommate is a force to be reckoned with - a no-nonsense girl who could put a professional nail artist to shame with her manicures. You could call her a serial dater I suppose, and we joked about it a lot.

"Hey girl! Did I tell you about this new dating app?" B asked.

"Another one? Sure you're ready after the last incident with that shady guy?" I joked.

"Ha, yeah, but this one is different – and I've already joined. Here, check it out," passing over her phone. "You should totally get on it too!"

"Eh, I dunno," I muttered in hesitation. "It seems legit, but remember the last time we convinced each other to try something new?"

"Oh God," B laughed out loud.

"You were so sore from crossfit. Sitting down was torture and your arms swelled so bad you couldn't fit your scrubs," I playfully reminded my roommate. "Maybe this weekend we can create a profile," I suggested. It has been over a year and a half since my last long-term relationship sank.

"Deal!" Clicking our wine glasses, B persisted on. "But just imagine, by this time next week, you could be sipping wine with your dream dude instead of watching it on TV," B stated.

As our conversation continued unfolding, a Facebook notification on my phone went off.

"I like your motorcycle," a friendly face messaged.

"Huh? How the hell should I respond to that?" I asked my roommate, forgetting about my recent riding posts. "Was he social media stalking me?"

Admittedly, I was intrigued. I thought a little flirting couldn't hurt, since he seemed completely different than my ex, which was the goal. He was cute, in a boyish kind of way, and I recognized his swanky smile from a party last summer.

"Thank you. I not only ride, I used to race," writing back with a winky face emoji. "Do you ride?"

Turns out he and I shared numerous mutual friends, which alleviated any creepy vibes.

"Wouldn't you like to know?" he replied.

We found ourselves chatting the rest of the night until a decision was made to meet in-person for a date the following Friday.

Unbeknownst to him, that motorcycle, that same damn crotch rocket that wrecked my previous relationship, was about to open the door for us.

On the evening of our first date, Mr. "I-Work-Out-At-5-PM" was running three hours late.

"Our flight is now delayed," he texted, keeping me in the loop.

Great, I thought, rolling my eyes.

Then another message buzzed in."Right when the plane landed, a co-worker insisted I drive him home as I was his only ride. Trust me, I was pissed, and told him I was finally meeting this girl for the first time."

I sighed a mix of frustration and amusement. "It's going to be later than expected. Do you still want me to come over?" he added.

By this point, I truly thought I was being stood up, despite his constant updates on the comedy of errors.

"Just my luck – and to think I was really excited to meet him," I said, lowering my head.

"Well, who knows if he'll show. But either way, we should get this party started," B exclaimed, pulling out a corkscrew and raising a glass with a mischievous grin.

I looked up and couldn't help but laugh. "Wine not?" I responded, lifting my own glass in a toast.

Just then, another text arrived. "On my way, finally. I swear, this has been a day from hell. Can't wait to see you."

I showed the text to my roommate. She smirked and said, "If he's half as determined as he sounds, he might just be worth the wait."

With a smile, I took another sip of wine. "Here's to hoping!"

A few hours later and a couple of bottles deep, I giggled my way downstairs to answer the light knock on my door. In the cool rain stood a handsome guy in a basic white t-shirt and jeans, his face freshly shaved, with a sheepish smile. There was a hint of apology in his hazel eyes as he leaned in for a hug.

"Hi, I'm Kyle," he said – as if I didn't know his name. I smiled and took a moment to appreciate the view.

His biceps were pretty nice, and he was taller than I expected. As he hugged me, it felt like being wrapped in a blanket of warmth and protection. This is nice, different I thought, feeling a bit dreamy from the wine.

"Hi there, come on in and leave your shoes here at the door," I eagerly requested, blushing as I ran back upstairs to give my roommate the secret nod of approval. B was still sitting on the kitchen counter as we often did.

Laughing out loud, with her perfectly manicured nails, she poured him a welcome drink. "You look thirsty!" she said, handing him a glass.

He came across as confident, mysterious, and free-spirited. From what I could tell, he seemed like a good person. The three of us exchanged stories and laughter for a short while, the initial worry melting away. No one had eaten dinner, as the original plan was to cook together.

"Is anybody else hungry besides me?" B asked, bouncing off the counter.

"Yes," I exclaimed, glancing at the clock. "It's late, and I'm not sure what's still open. But let's see."

"Yeah, there was no time for me to eat. I could go for any food at this point," Kyle stated with a twist of humor.

The three of us hurried downstairs, threw our shoes on, and ran outside to Kyle's gray-blue Ford Taurus. Buffalo Wild Wings was calling our names. Even in the rain, the first thing I noticed were the tiny rust patches along the wheel well. Chivalry hadn't died yet, as he opened the passenger side door for me to climb inside.

"Nice car," I said with a smile, trying to ignore the rust spots.

"Thanks," he replied with a grin. "She's a classic."

As I settled in, the second thing I noticed was the little rubber chicken strangely hanging out of the air vent. Maybe this guy is not so vanilla after all? I thought, specifically recalling a recent conversation with my best friend Liz. The plan was to date someone unlike all my ex's. So far he was hitting the mark.

B, hopping into the backseat, immediately noticed the chicken too. "What's with the rubber chicken?" she asked, barely stifling a laugh.

He chuckled. "Oh, that was a pep rally gift from the football cheerleaders back in college."

I raised an eyebrow, intrigued.

"So, Buffalo Wild Wings, huh? Are you a spicy wings kind of guy?" I asked.

He glanced over at me with a smirk. "Nope! Just mild with buffalo sauce. I had a bad experience with a friend and the blazin' wing challenge a while back. You?"

"I prefer boneless - maybe teriyaki," I said confidently.

B chimed in from the back, "Sounds like none of us will be doing the wing challenge."

We all laughed – enjoying each other's company.

After some much needed food, we all arrived back at my condo. It was too late for Kyle to make the two-hour trek home.

He glanced at the time, then at the oversized couch. "I guess this is me for the night," he suggested, making himself comfortable.

I watched him struggle with the cushions and laughed. "You know, the bed has more space and fewer lumps."

He looked up, surprised. "Are you sure?"

"Absolutely," I said, smiling and waving him into my bedroom.

As he settled beside me in bed, I couldn't help but to indulge in my quickly growing feelings.

"Honestly, I'm glad you stayed," our eyes met. He leaned in, his lips brushing mine, and we shared our first kiss.

My heart felt as light as a feather.

It was then I realized that even though I hadn't been in a romantic relationship with someone in a while – I was never actually single.

We are always in a relationship with ourselves.

So my friends, stay committed to yourself. Stay committed to evolving and the right person will come along.

CHAPTER 9

Harbor of Hearts

*"You are the one that possesses the keys to your being.
You carry the passport to your own happiness."*
—Diane von Furstenberg

A year flew by and I could hardly believe it. The long drives and late night conversations would come to an end, as Kyle and I decided it was time to take the next step and move in together. I transferred my employment where I worked as a school director, and we quickly settled into his duplex.

It was perfect for us – well, almost.

"You know," I said one evening, "we're practically outgrowing this space already...," nudging him playfully.

"Yea, I know..." he replied in a sarcastic tone.

With the economy doing well, we knew it was a good time to sell my condo, which I had been renting out. The plan was to use the money from the sale for a land payment to build our own home in a community halfway between our jobs.

The decision was bittersweet.

The day had arrived when I had to say goodbye to my condo – the first property I ever owned, the space that provided comfort and triumph after much devastation. Kyle and I met my realtor in the kitchen, ready for the farewell signing.

As we went through the paperwork, Kyle stood in the corner, absorbed in his cell phone. I tried to keep my annoyance in check, smiling at the realtor, who was being incredibly encouraging.

"This is such a great move for you," he said warmly. "The market is perfect right now, and you'll make a great profit."

"Thanks," I replied, genuinely appreciating his support. "It's definitely time."

Just before my John Handcock, I took one last stroll around memory lane. I wandered through the rooms, each one echoing with memories – the late-night binge sessions, the celebratory dinners, the quiet moments of reflection.

In the corner of the kitchen, Kyle was still glued to his phone, tapping away. "Hey, we're about to sign. Hello? What are you doing? Get off your phone," I called out, rolling my eyes while trying to sound more cheerful than annoyed.

"Uh-huh, just a second," he mumbled, not looking up.

I laughed nervously, wiping away a tear and turning back to the realtor. "Sorry, he's working on something important. Timing, right?"

The realtor gave a sympathetic smile. "It's a big day for both of you."

I nodded, taking a deep breath. "Yeah, it's bittersweet, but I'm ready for it."

Finally, Kyle looked up and walked over to the table. "Sorry, I just had to finish something. You okay?"

"Yeah," I said, forcing a smile. "Let's do this."

An anchor brought my mind and body right back into the feelings of mistrust that stemmed from my ex's.

Five minutes and a few signed documents later, the deal was done.

"Well, that's it. Congratulations, Stephanie," my realtor said kindly. "Let me know if there's anything else I can help you with in the future – business or friend-wise."

"Thank you so much," I replied, grateful for his support over the years.

Before departing the premises, the only remaining task was the final cleaning.

"I'll wipe the entryway windows while you, Handyman, re-check the bedrooms," I suggested.

"Sure thing, I'll go grab the screwdriver out of the car," Kyle agreed, frantically exiting.

It was getting late. My stomach was growling in hunger, as I stomped my way back downstairs to answer the knock at the door. "What took him so long? He must have locked himself out," I mumbled while opening the door.

In the cool rain, a familiar stranger stood, dressed in a basic white t-shirt, jeans, a handsome 5 o'clock shadow and a sheepish smile. There was a hint of enthusiasm in his hazel eyes.

"Hi. Does this look familiar?" he asked awkwardly.

I turned sideways with my paper towel, on a mission to tidy the small square window panels so we could finally go to dinner. "Kind of like the first time we—"

Before I could finish the sentence, Kyle dropped to one knee and opened a small red box. Everything blurred around me.

I didn't even notice the video camera in the corner or the lovely bottle of champagne hidden in the bushes.

Kyle never looked so sexy. I feel bad for scolding him while he prepared to ask for my hand, I thought to myself.

Am I crying or is that the rain? Wait, what is he saying? This is a big decision. I love him, so of course I will say yes.

Crap, I'm not listening, the voice in my head wouldn't shut up. At least I forgot about how hungry I was.

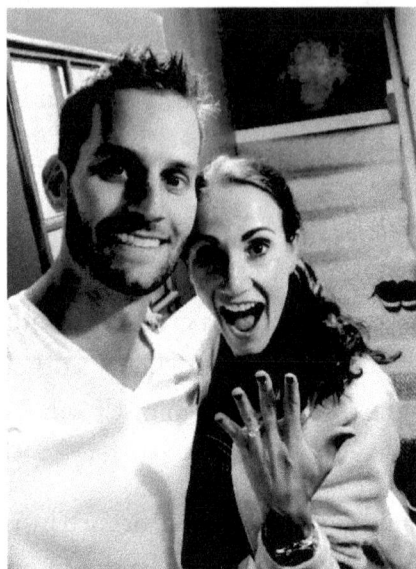

"Yes," I yelled before accepting the diamond and kissing my fiancé!

CHAPTER 10

Tying the Knot

"Encouraging someone to be entirely themselves is the loudest way to love them" —Kalen Dion

---

Standing at the top of the cement stairs of the Grand Geneva Resort, I felt the moment settle into my chest in the most intense way.

Excited for the biggest day of my life, I was also feeling the nerves kicking in as our large wedding party exited the building doors.

"Where's my personal attendant? Is it time already? How's my make-up?"

Tears began forming in my freshly painted eyes, blurring my vision. "Are my eyelashes falling off?" I muttered, trying to distract myself with humor as my hands trembled. "Oh my gosh, get it together, Stephanie," I asserted out loud, a bit more forcefully than intended.

My wedding planner, noticing my distress, stepped beside me and gently touched my shoulder. "You're doing great," she said soothingly. "Your makeup is flawless, and your eyelashes are fine. Just take a deep breath."

So I took a deep breath, trying to steady myself. "Thank you," I whispered, still feeling the flutter of nerves.

As the melody of Hayley Reinhart's "I Can't Help Falling in Love" filled the air, my heart began racing. The ceremony was starting on time, and I didn't feel as prepared as I thought I would.

The planner smiled reassuringly. "Okay, Stephanie, this is your big day – ready here we go."

Nodding, I took another deep breath.

And then I reflected back on the incredible life Kyle and I had been building since the beginning. From the first message I received about my motorcycle that outlasted the sinking ship, to the hand-written vows we would read to each other, every terrible relationship, even the ones I didn't include in this book, led me to this very moment.

But it wasn't just the romantic relationships that shaped me—it was the complicated ones, too. The messy, unresolved parts of my past that, in their own way, had also brought me here.

My rose gold studded heels and I took the first step together.

My dress, a stunning white gown adorned with countless sparkling beads, shimmered in the sunlight that peeked through the clouds. Nearing the middle of the staircase, a tug on my hair made me wonder if someone had accidentally stepped on my long veil. But it didn't matter, I had to keep moving. Turns out, the veil flowing down my back lifted in a gust of wind that seemed to come at the picture perfect time. The photographer captured it all beautifully.

At the bottom of the stairs, my father stood waiting.

The first man who ever loved me. The first man in my life who had agreed to give my hand to the last.

There hadn't always been sunshine between us. It felt like dad and I had a strained relationship for years, one that neither of us seemed capable of fixing. That high school phone call cut me deep. I never thought I would measure up. I never thought I was "good enough." And I carried that weight for a long time – until the night I graduated from college.

After celebrating with drinks at a bar, Dad and I sat until the early hours of the morning, talking in a way we never had before. I finally told him how much his harshness hurt me, how sincerely I craved his approval and how I always felt like I wasn't enough for him. He sat quietly, his eyes focused somewhere far away, before finally telling me the truth I had longed to hear: he was proud of me.

Dad was proud of the woman I had become.

He also admitted that sometimes I reminded him of my mother. I hadn't realized how much unresolved pain he carried, how it influenced the way he viewed me. That night, we mended something broken between us. The gap began closing, and it was like we both could breathe again.

Standing here now, as he waited to walk me down the aisle, his smile was peaceful. His beaming blue eyes, filled with pride and love, gave me the strength I needed. He extended his arm, and I took it, feeling a sense of calm as we locked elbows.

"Ready?" he asked softly, his voice steady and reassuring.

"As I'll ever be," I whispered, my voice thick with emotion.

Together, we turned the corner and began the long walk down the grass aisle sprinkled with light pink flower petals. I glanced at my dad and whispered, "You know what they say about the grass being greener on the other side?"

He looked at me, slightly puzzled. "Huh?"

I grinned, squeezing his arm. "Never mind," I said, shaking my head with a smile. As we continued walking, I couldn't help but think, Well, this grass is definitely the greenest I've ever seen – right where I'm walking.

Elegant blush bows hung on the side of the white chairs, filled with family and friends smiling. Their faces were glowing with happiness and excitement – and many using the programs I created, too.

But not everyone I loved was in attendance. My younger brother, who should have been standing with the groomsmen, was absent. I truly wished that he could be there for me today. But he couldn't, because he was in jail – on a path that had taken him far from the light I prayed he would one day find again.

I missed him.

I missed the version of him I once knew when we were kids, before life pulled him into darkness. My heart hurt knowing how far he was from this beautiful day, both physically and emotionally. But I hadn't given up hope. I still prayed that he would find his way back to himself, and to the love he deserved.

Even today, I have that hope for him...

And then our eyes met. My handsome husband-to-be, standing at the end of the aisle in his navy-blue suit, white shirt, and signature scruffy beard. Seeing him there waiting proudly, filled my heart with indescribable joy.

Surrounding him were our groomsmen and bridesmaids, each one a pillar of our shared history and future. My father shook Kyle's hand with the understanding, "take care of her forever," before lightly placing his hand on the swell of my back and pushing me forward.

It wasn't long before we mixed sands, shared vows, and officially tied the knot.

The world around us seemed to blur, leaving only the two of us in the perfect, shared space.

I felt an overwhelming sense of gratitude.

Gratitude for the journey that had brought me here.

Gratitude for the man who stood beside me.

Gratitude for the new chapter we were about to begin together. "We do!"

Love is a funny thing. And although I fell in love with Kyle, the truth is I hadn't completely fallen in love with myself yet.

In the end, you realize it's just you. No one is coming to save you. No one can lift you up like you can. And no one can overcome the experiences you went through. It will always be you.

So if you can, find someone who will help you return to the love within yourself, over and over again. When you love yourself deeply, you bring the best version of yourself to every relationship. You become unstoppable.

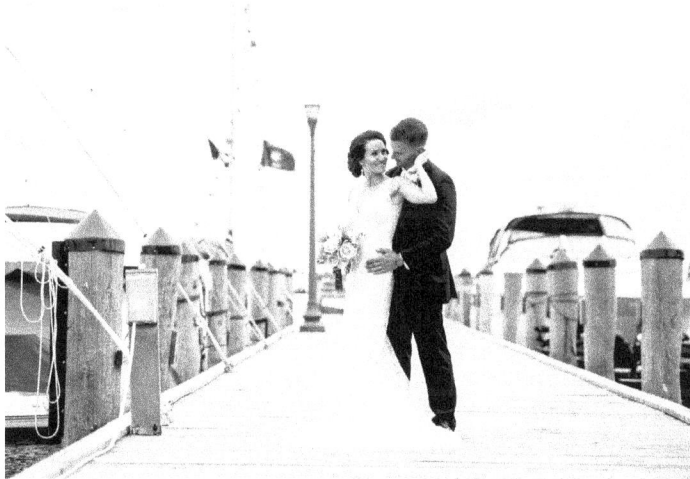

This Nauti Girl committed to Kyle – and to navigating my naked truth.

CHAPTER 11

SEAS the Day

"A journey toward trauma healing and self-worth begins with the willingness to hold a vision for new ways of living" —Stephanie Kraemer

---

There I was – watching my husband gulp down his reheated coffee from his "World's Best Husband" mug. Meanwhile, I was unpacking a bag of complaints about my work in healthcare. I moaned about the communal chaos that seemed to plague every team and then ranted about anything and everything I could word-vomit that morning.

"She should get fired and stop using excuses to stay employed." "I should just tell the director what's really going on!" "She should never have come back." "Or maybe I should leave cat shit on her porch?" I was shoulding all over myself again!

Rejecting the notion that I was to blame for anything, yet my shoulders were carrying the weight of the Titanic. We all know how that ship sailed – or didn't!

My toxic co-worker's attitude for any type of collaboration was lost. It wasn't just her knack for microaggressions that had me distressed on the daily. While navigating the trenches of workplace toxicity, the whole world seemed to be teetering on edge amidst a pandemic.

It was much more.

It felt bigger, heavier, like a tidal wave of powerlessness that has been building over time, now crashing in harder with each passing moment. I couldn't breathe – my eyes clouded with a misty haze.

Back in the kitchen, I stood silently demanding my husband to divulge the magic solutions to my "problems" and anger. He sat there, the epitome of patience, nodding along and sipping his elixir of sanity. His silence felt foolishly unjustified.

For the love of God, speak, I thought to myself while craving validation.

Absurdly, I wanted him to join me in the trenches and suffer alongside. I wanted him to endorse the take-down of this person. I wanted him to confirm my feelings. Unable to keep my mouth shut, I impulsively insisted he say–anything–to lift my spirits.

"Are you just going to sit there and ignore me? Say something, ugh!" The audacity of desperation!

Moments later, he chimed in with a sarcastic twist on my life's mantra, "seize the day, Steph," his tone wet with playful mockery. I wanted to laugh, but instead lightly slapped his shoulder. I replied back, "carpe this diem!" as a grin snuck its way onto my face.

I didn't know what else to say because somehow, he was already right, airing my buried beliefs.

He has a way of creating space for me to think. My husband knows me, the raw, unfiltered version.

Of course, the actual answers in pursuance were not as simple as Carpe Diem, or "seize the day" in Latin. But the witty comment stopped my train of thought dead in my tracks.

As my husband stood up from the table, he said something along the lines of "I don't know exactly what to tell you. But, when you look back at life, what are you going to regret more – working unhappily for an organization while building somebody else's dreams, or quitting and building your own? Go write your book or do what you want – but 'quit' complaining and make a decision."

With his walk-away tactic, and "I'm here for you" vibe, he left me pondering his words, a mix of tough love and unwavering support – a classic move from the book of husband wisdom.

Sure, I wished for a one-way ticket to hell for my co-worker. But at the same time, I needed to uncover why her actions and behaviors felt so provoking. I needed to think and reflect.

Admittedly, I also needed a shower!

Standing within the shiny, hexagon-tiled enclosure, a flood of old memories started to surface. The sudden click of the glass door closing startled me as I reached to adjust the lever. Cool water, then warmth sprinkled over my bare skin. I was struggling to quiet the inner conflicts, feeling the weight of my own contradictions pressing in. Different aspects of my identity were demanding attention, just yearning to be acknowledged and understood.

Why haven't I moved past these experiences despite my previous efforts, I wondered? What the heck is happening and why wasn't I fixed? Questioning the remnants of childhood trauma that were clearly still influencing various facets of my life.

So much trauma, so little recovery.

Thinking out loud, afterall the self-care I've done, does anyone actually heal?

Maybe what they've been teaching us is a lie?

The goal is not to fix ourselves because we are not broken.

Maybe we simply are not meant to ever fully heal?

Like those living with alcoholism – maybe we are all traumaholics? Maybe we learn to live with our trauma every day?

As a self-appointed life-long learner, I now believe that when things happen, we create the meaning; the reason; the lesson. It was time to come clean – to wash the stains I perpetually held on to.

Turning off the shower, I slowly stepped out, careful not to slip on a cat or two. The room was foggy, forgetting to turn on the fan as I often do. Wiping the condensation from the mirror, our eyes met. There she was, young Stephanie starring back.

Drenched in goddamn dread, standing naked, truth dripping from the seams of my soul.

I asked myself, What have I done by denying these feelings in my old self for so long? When was the last time I asked myself what I wanted rather than what the world wanted from me?

I was finally sitting with my emotions, rather than drowning in them.

Despite the official day off from work, I put on my house robe, walked downstairs to my nautical-themed home office and settled into my swivel chair. My identity was woven with a commitment to service, but also defined by my role as a dedicated team player, always striving to exceed expectations.

Sitting in silence, it was difficult to drown out the voices in my head.

Hang in there, Stephanie!

You are such an asset!

Don't quit just yet. Things will get better!

Ugh, what a shame. You don't deserve this!

Deserve, thinking out loud. *What do I deserve?*

Surrendering to the unknown was a new feeling, met with discomfort and grief.

You see, it wasn't that long ago my supervisor Heidi and I hit the pavement for a lunch break stroll outside. As health-conscious humans, we often took walking meetings to think clearly and get our steps in. Our professional business attire didn't matter, as we both kept extra sneakers at the office.

I recall a specific conversation, as the wind whipped my boss's brunette hair around.

"I have to be completely transparent with you regarding my feelings about my colleague," I stated, while biting the inside of my cheek. Although this was not the first conversation we were having about the toxic situation, something in me was changing. Tensions had been brewing as I found myself at more than odds with a certain co-worker. "Ugh. She's so manipulative. I constantly feel undermined during team meetings and presentations – her subtle jabs hidden behind her snaky smile and stolen ideas! I'm so over it," tasting my bitterness and warning, "week after week, I feel my confidence diminishing and my disgust rising."

As we continued walking, Heidi calmly replied, "First off, I'm so sorry you are going through all of this. I understand why you feel the way you do and I'm here for you. You are a valued member of the team. The last thing I want is to see you leave."

My heart started to race, and my shoulders became tense. I needed to vent and knew this would be a safe channel to do so, to express what I experienced every day in the workplace due to this one individual.

"My anxiety, anger and low self-worth anchors have begun taking control. I appreciate you saying what you did. But what about the recent meeting," I questioned, reminding Heidi about the mask slip, revealing a glimpse of my co-workers true nature. "She exploded, yelling, swearing and finger pointing," shocking us into silence. Her volatile temper left a lingering tension in the air.

"I guess I'm just not sure at what point my mental health and dreams become more important. I don't know what to do anymore," I emphasized as my eyes slowly filled with water.

"You just have to trust me. We are doing everything we can. I wish I could say more," Heidi added.

I could hear the sincerity in her voice. Her kindness and compassion always present. Though her supportive demeanor helped release some stress that had been building up, I also knew human resources limited her ability to assist me further.

"I don't understand why you can't fire her. I worked in HR; I know the game. Nineteen policy violations, including swearing at a supervisor, should be grounds for immediate termination," I exclaimed!

"I do not want to talk badly about people. I hear you Stephanie; I really do. It's not that simple though."

"Why not?" now sounding like a whiny two-year-old.

"There is a process we must go through. And that's all I can say. You just have to trust me."

My cat jumped on my lap, waking me from the daydream. But with the conversation on the top of my mind, I was spinning in my head, and in the chair.

Why do I feel like Tom Hanks in Cast Away?

For a woman with a larger-than-life personality, what the hell happened to me? How did I get here?

"Is this really the right move?" I muttered to myself, doubts creeping back in like unwelcome guests. "Maybe I'm making a mistake if I quit."

The knots in my stomach tightened as the fear of letting others down grew. Who was I looking to receive permission from – and why do I need permission at all?

Do I have the right to quit – I mean, of course I do? I have the right to be who I want, have whatever I want in life… don't I? As the words hung in the air, my thoughts echoed back like whispers of uncertainty.

In my various careers over the years, I always took pride in being an excellent employee and colleague. I've seen plenty of adults who just coast by, doing the bare minimum for a paycheck. Not me. That has never been who I am. Accountability has always been a core value, and I couldn't shake the worry of who would step up to handle all the tasks and projects I'd leave behind?

Who will ensure the volunteers feel appreciated? Who will facilitate the upcoming training? And what about the new campaign we are supposed to be launching this year?

Each responsibility felt like a piece of my commitment to excellence. The last thing I wanted was to let anyone down or face failure. But even as I grappled with these concerns, I knew that accountability also meant taking ownership of my choices, even if they led to uncertainty.

Ever since I was fourteen years old, I've held a job and harbored a strong aversion to laziness. I've poured my heart and soul into my work, earning degrees and advancing in my careers to prove my worth. For me, a reliable nine-to-five wasn't just a means of earning a living; it was a testament to my dedication and capabilities.

It was a way to prove my worth to the world.

Yet, despite my efforts, the nagging feeling of powerlessness and instability loomed at large.

It's the limiting beliefs that keep us small.

"Am I even worthy of healing?" I grumbled to myself. "How dare I prioritize my own needs over others'. Why do I feel so… guilty?"

I could practically hear the judgmental voices of my friends and family echoing in my head. "Must be nice to not have to work," they sneered. "Oh, what are you doing today, sleeping?" they scoffed. "Who does she think she is, a gold digger?" The barrage of criticism felt like daggers to my already fragile sense of self-worth.

It's the limiting beliefs that keep us small.

Desperate for validation of my seemingly selfish decision, I scanned the room in a game of "I Spy," searching for anything to confirm its validity. And then, I saw it – mocked by my husband earlier this morning – a seemingly trivial sign and personal motto, "seize the day." What I hadn't shared was the clever twist in its spelling, matching the room's maritime theme: "Seas" the Day!

Suddenly, it wasn't just a motto anymore; it emerged as a powerful affirmation for the transformative journey I was embarking upon.

I hit send, submitting my letter of resignation.

CHAPTER 12

Self-Awareness

"It isn't where you came from; it's where you're going that counts." —Ella Fitzgerald

---

Rarely do we heal by accident.

Healing is so hard because it's a constant battle between your inner child, who's scared and just wants safety; your inner teenager who's angry and just wants justice; and your adult self, who is tired and just wants peace.

It was one of those stale evenings when I didn't feel like socializing, and the allure of staying in was irresistible. Slipping into my comfiest loungewear, I poured myself a generous, Stephanie sized glass of liquid therapy and settled onto the couch cushions. My two feline friends, Malibu and Bailey, appeared as if on cue. Always eager for cuddles, their soft purrs added to the unwind. The hubby was working late, which made it a perfect chick-flick kind of night. "You're not drinking alone if your cats are home," I thought outloud. Little did I know, my evening of Netflix and chill would turn into a crash course in self-awareness.

While indulging in the comfort of my surroundings, I found myself drawn to a familiar storyline on the screen. The main character, a middle-aged woman dealing with her own demons, mirrored the complexities of my own life in ways I hadn't expected. In one scene, she turned to her therapist and asked something like: "Isn't there a point in my journey where I'm supposed to trust myself?"

According to Hollywood's version of a shrink, "you can't trust the person you are until you stop denying the person you once were."

I found myself nodding along, engaged with an empty wine glass and a couple judgemental stares.

The therapist went on, "embracing all parts of ourselves, including our past, is essential for developing genuine self-trust and love. Only when we acknowledge and integrate our past can we truly appreciate and trust ourselves."

It was as though all three of us were pondering the meaning of life, love, and the pursuit of a clean litter box. Holy mic drop, kitties. "Self-awareness isn't about having all the answers; it's about embracing the messy, complicated, imperfect humanness that we are."

Humaning is hard!

Throwing the blanket aside, I made my way downstairs to retrieve my journal. The urgency of the message compelled me to put pen to paper. It felt as though it held significance not only for me in the present, but also for sharing with others in the future.

Hurrying back upstairs to the couch, I wrote these words: "Befriend the grief! Befriend the messy!"

As the credits rolled on the screen, the therapist's words continued on replay. When we begin the process of understanding ourselves and making peace with our past, we learn to become self-aware.

Self-awareness grows appreciation for the now, and how far we've come.

By denying or neglecting our past experiences, we hinder our ability to develop genuine trust and self-worth.

Have you ever taken a moment to sit and think about yourself? You know, wondered why you act a certain way or second-guessed your feelings or beliefs? No? Don't worry, you're not alone. It seems like most people do not give themselves that much scrutiny. People tend to search for answers on the outside versus looking within.

Maybe not so secretly, I have always been drawn to people who embrace their uniqueness – the purple cows, the dreamers, the wild ones, and the creatives. These are the individuals who march to the beat of their own drum, unswayed by the pressures of conformity or groupthink. Interestingly, my dad used to be a drummer. I guess my mom couldn't resist the rhythm of love. Ha!

In my non-expert, non-therapist opinion, what sets these people apart is their willingness to reflect upon their actions. They are able to ask questions and be curious when anchors arise.

Beginning a healing journey means surrendering to the parts of ourselves that weigh heavy, acknowledging those anchors holding us back. This process involves facing our trauma and grief head-on and understanding that it is a part of us. By befriending grief, we can learn to navigate its depths, allowing it to coexist with us.

Admit the bullshit! Then give it a hug.

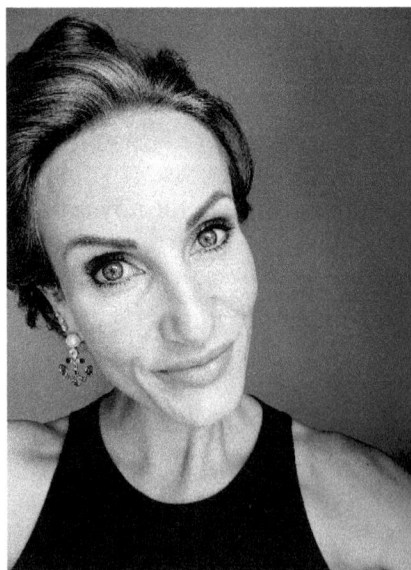

Admitting, rather than avoiding, transforms our relationship with trauma, helping us find strength and resilience in the process.

A few days later, hubby was working late again, I came across a Tony Robbins workshop ad on my phone. Rather, the ad found me. Usually, I'd swipe past the plethora of self-help pitches with a smirk, but something about this one made me pause. Maybe it was the hypnotic cadence of Tony's words, as they seemed to pierce through my screen and straight into my soul.

Either way, I found myself clicking on the link and, before I knew it, signing up for the workshop.

Day one of the workshop was all about self-awareness and breaking through. Tony, with his booming voice and infectious energy, challenged us to dive deep into our own minds with questions like "why are you here," and "what's prevented you from creating your extraordinary life?"

We spent hours reflecting and writing. And no, I do not receive commission from sharing this information.

Paying close attention to my emotions, I began realizing all the time I've spent drifting in the shallow waters of my consciousness, avoiding the deeper darker currents of my true self. Curiosity was bubbling within me. Tony said something like, "you can't heal what you won't reveal," and it hit me like a tidal wave. But what I heard was, "admit the bullshit, Steph."

You can't change what you don't acknowledge – and I was ready to face whatever was needed.

Tony's exercises pushed me to confront these emotions and questions head-on. I closed my eyes and let his words guide me. It felt like the permission I needed to pause.

It felt like the permission I needed to forgive myself for all the times I didn't trust my intuition – my gut. We all carry those moments, don't we? Those whispers from our inner voice that we pushed aside, only to find ourselves nursing a bruised ego later.

Permission to come aboard!

Memories surfaced, some murky and others crystal clear, each one a piece of the puzzle that formed my identity. What I began realizing is that I already possessed the resources needed for healing.

Rather than looking back with regret, I began finding forgiveness for past versions of myself who ignored the red flags – versions who stayed in shitty situations. I found forgiveness for dimming my own light – for not speaking my truth.

Forgiveness is not erasing the past, but choosing to learn from it without being chained to it.

The act of self-forgiveness is also the act of becoming self-aware.

Healing begins and ends with us, not other people. We control our emotions so if we can't change a situation, we need to change our perception of it. I began recognizing patterns in my reactions and choices, and knew I had to keep exploring.

When triggered and anchors reveal themselves, emotions are raw, often heightened to the point they cloud your ability to think clearly. Remember my relationship and robbery story – who did I call? Nope, not the ghostbusters, but my ex. The very same ex who contributed to the trauma I experienced. Yikes. Zero self-awareness.

Old keys do not unlock new doors.

In the midst of our fast-paced lives, we are often taught how to do – how to accomplish. Yet, we seldom learn the art of pausing to connect with our inner selves or to reflect before moving forward.

So when a situation creates an anchor for you, and you too feel stuck in the muck, I encourage – in fact, I give you permission to pause – and to forgive. Don't call your ex!

By working on our healing through self-awareness first, we begin stripping away the layers, the good, bad and messy in between, covering the core of who we are. This is where we begin learning how our past affects us now, shaping how we see things, relate to others, and handle challenges.

And it's not just about the big stuff either, like facing fears or confronting painful memories. It's also about those little moments of noticing – like realizing when something feels "off" or understanding why we react certain ways in particular situations.

Through my journey of self-awareness, I've come to realize that I reached out to Jason because I had already exposed my vulnerability. And while I honor that part of my past, if faced with the same situation today, I'd choose differently.

Rather than calling my ex, I'd allow myself space to let the lack of power and the sadness subside before reacting.

Never let boredom, loneliness or temporary suffering be the reason you go back to people, places, or circumstances that weighed you down in the first place.

That feeling of powerlessness was one of the biggest contributors to staying in sinking relationships, not to mention delaying my own healing journey.

But where focus goes, energy flows.

The more I delve into my thoughts and emotional turbulence, the more I witness them rise to the surface to be adjusted. This deep introspection and willingness to engage with my internal "instruments" feels incredibly empowering.

While developing self-awareness won't exclusively – or completely – heal trauma, it serves as a crucial starting point.

By ensuring that our internal compass functions accurately, we can steer ourselves with greater confidence, equipped with the insight needed to face challenges that come our way.

You see, after that final kiss with Jason, I bet my friends I'd miss him. Turns out, I missed me more!

CHAPTER 13
Exploring Belief Systems

"There comes a point where we need to stop just pulling people out of the river. We need to go upstream and find out why they're falling in."
—Desmond Tutu

As I approach the Spa entrance, the stresses of the outside world begin to melt away. The renovated building, modern yet inviting, exudes a sense of tranquility with its clean lines and natural materials. It's been a minute since I've treated myself.

Walking in, the lobby is bathed in natural light streaming through large windows near a small shopping area filled with soaps and souvenirs. I just love the scent of lavender and eucalyptus. Promptly, I am greeted by the friendly, soft-spoken receptionist whose smile is pleasant. She speaks in hushed tones, a good reminder for my loudmouth self to dial it down a notch.

"Good morning and welcome. I can assist you over here. Have you been with us before?"

"Hi there. Yes I have," I grinned proudly.

"Are you checking in for an appointment today?"

"Actually, this time I'm only utilizing the day pass with amenities. My name is Stephanie Kraemer."

As the receptionist efficiently checks me in, I notice the subtle background music – gentle, and perfectly tuned to calm the mind and the fierce typing skills in front of me. I don't know about you, but quieting the noise in my head is a very difficult process. My goal for the day was relaxation. My goal for the year was to let go of things no longer serving me; people, experiences and thoughts. I wished myself luck!

On the other side of the building was the swim up bar pool with 84-degree water and plenty of private conversation coves for this chatty Kathy. Wearing my swimsuit, towel-robe and sandals, I squeaked my way over and planted myself tight to the bar to strike up a conversation with the mocktail mixologist.

"Hello. What can I get for you today?" asked the waiter.

"Hi. I'd like the Fizzy Figgy Tea, please."

The cheerful young man eager to please, responded with a smile, "coming right up! Oh, have you tried our new menu? We have some amazing snacks that pair perfectly with our drinks."

"No, I haven't. What do you recommend?" I asked, glancing at the waterproof menu he handed me. Old habits die hard – I still found myself reading menus from left to right.

"I'd recommend the ahi tuna bowl; it's fresh and delicious!"

"Oh, that sounds perfect. I'll take one of those too," I replied. "Thanks!"

As I peered over to another woman sitting down from me, I noticed her drink.

"Oh, and what's that you're sipping on?" I asked, curiosity piqued.

The woman, a stylish brunette with a welcoming smile, chimed in, "It's the Rose Refresher. You should try it!"

"That was my grandmother's name. I guess I'll have to – thanks!" I replied enthusiastically. Looking back over to the bartender, he nodded while overhearing our conversation.

It didn't take long for the woman and I to begin our banter. At first, it was the usual: our names, where we were from, and what we did for work.

"Well, I recently left my job in healthcare and decided to write a book," I shared, feeling a sense of liberation as I spoke the words out loud.

"That's amazing!" she exclaimed, her eyes lighting up. "What's your book about?"

The conversation flowed naturally. And just as the woman finished her early lunch, I mumbled, "Clean plate club."

She looked up, a quizzical smile forming. "Did you just say 'clean plate club'?"

"Sometimes I open my mouth and my mother comes out," I responded with a laugh.

"Oh, I know that feeling all too well," she chuckled. "My mom used to say that all the time."

"Would she follow it up with a guilt trip down 'you know there are starving children in the world' lane, too?"

I had no idea my subtle comment would send me spiraling into one of my manic episodes – obsessing over a topic.

The woman nodded knowingly. "My grandmother was a stickler for the clean plate club. Sometimes it even became a competition of who could finish their food the fastest," the woman discussed.

It's funny how these little sayings stick with us, reflecting the beliefs of previous generations.

"You know, sometimes I think about all those uneaten vegetables, and I feel like I should apologize to them."

"Right?" I said, grinning. "What did they ever do to deserve being shoved around a plate?"

We both laughed, sipping our drinks, the humor lightening the conversation. It was a relief to find someone who understood the strange power of these ingrained beliefs. I felt a sense of camaraderie and understanding.

"To the leave-a-bite club!" she echoed, clinking her plastic glass against mine.

Our conversation had taken an unexpected turn, but it was a reminder of how deeply our beliefs are embedded in us, and how they can shape our thoughts and actions in the most surprising ways.

After finishing my food, we said our Wisconsin goodbyes and I splashed my way over to one of the sandstone formation coves. "Great," I mused, I'm at a luxurious spa, and here I am obsessing over leftover mashed potatoes from 1992, drowning myself in my thoughts.

Suddenly, I felt the "lack anchor" pulling me down.

"This is the shit that keeps me up at night," I thought out loud.

Sitting there, I recalled many childhood dinner conversations. My brothers and I couldn't leave the table until all three slots of food were eaten. No excuses were accepted because, after all, "there were starving children in other countries."

Have you ever just sat, chewing on your thoughts, wondering how you became... you? Do you ever question your personality or what factors have influenced your current beliefs about yourself and the world? I tend to think about this stuff all too often.

Do you ever wonder how much of your behavior is a result of those early experiences? How many of your beliefs are inherited rather than chosen?

For me, the "scarcity mentality" I learned early on manifested into not being enough or deserving, keeping me in unhealthy patterns. Additionally, the feeling of powerlessness carried into adolescence and beyond, influencing many thoughts and decisions.

What patterns have you noticed in your own life that might trace back to your early experiences? How do these patterns shape your interactions and choices today?

My mind shifted from mashed potatoes to something even messier.

I still hate, and hesitate, saying the word – the "R" word. Gross.

When it comes to exploring belief systems, it can be tricky to reveal the thoughts, words, and beliefs that run deep within us.

Thoughts are the building blocks of who we are.

Thoughts externalized become our words. And our words become powerful actions and behaviors, which ultimately shape the outcome of our lives.

Our thoughts are those stories we create in our minds that no one else sees – our own private soap operas. Although some thoughts can seem very real, they don't technically exist outside of ourselves – unless we turn them into reality.

The great thing about thoughts; you own yours, and I own mine!

No one can force us to think anything, which means we can change our thoughts whenever we want. It's like having a remote control for your brain! Except for me, there's no off button.

The idea of thoughts is incredibly powerful. According to experts, we have about 60,000 thoughts per day, and 90% of them are repetitive. This means the more we think about something, the more it becomes hard-wired into our memories, and the more it becomes who we are.

Therefore, we do not just experience life, but rather, we experience the life we continually focus on.

Our thoughts are deeply influenced by our perceptions and can either be detrimental or empowering. Think about one belief you are holding on to right now. It may be that you can't achieve your health goal or quit your 9-5. Or it may be that you are qualified for the job promotion, and you are worthy of having a loving relationship. Regardless of what you believe, you are correct.

But first... perception.

Perceptions are like the lenses of sunglasses through which we view the outside world. They shape our thoughts and color our reality.

Remember, where our focus goes, energy flows!

By zooming in on certain details, experiences, or ideas, we fuel the quality of our thoughts that become central to who we are. Think of your perception as a gatekeeper to your mind. They decide what is fed and then becomes embedded into your thoughts.

Garbage in, garbage out!

If we consume negative content, engage in toxic conversations, or follow draining social media channels, our thoughts will mirror that negativity. But surround yourself with positive people, enriching content, and supportive relationships, our thoughts will flourish.

Choose your mental diet wisely, my friends.

What are you watching on television or scrolling on your phone? Who are you surrounding yourself with? In a room full of opportunities, would they say your name? What does your work environment feel like?

All of this matters because our choices in the external world can shape and influence our internal world. By being mindful of what we consume, who we spend time with, and the environments we create, we can actively steer our thoughts towards more positive belief systems.

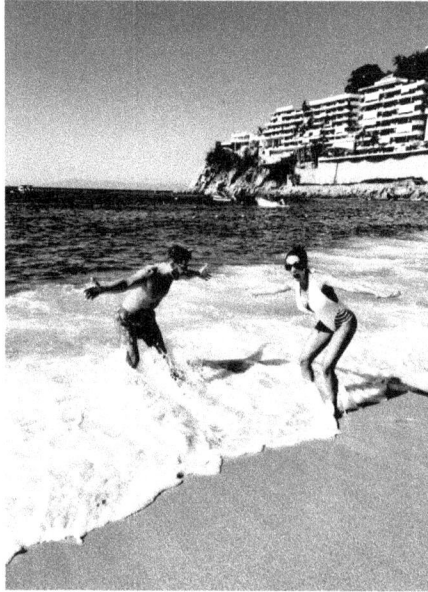

Words

"The most powerful words in the universe are the words you say to yourself" —Marie Forleo

Now, let's transition to how these thoughts manifest in our daily lives. Our thoughts are the precursors to our words. What we consistently think about eventually finds its way into our speech. When you think positively, your words reflect that positivity, and when you harbor negative thoughts, it shows in your language.

Power is in the tongue.

Words influence our actions and behaviors. They can uplift and inspire, or discourage and deflate.

Speak life into yourself!

Imagine a simple phrase like, "I can do this," "I am beautiful and worthy," or "I am enough." If these thoughts become a regular part of your internal dialogue (I keep sticky notes on my mirror), they transform into your spoken words. These words then influence your belief systems and ultimately your actions.

Conversely, repeatedly thinking and saying, "I can't do this," can trap you in a cycle of inaction and self-sabotage. It's like having a note saying "NOPE" stuck to your forehead – definitely not the vibe we're going for!

Words are like little affirmations that we broadcast to ourselves and to the world. They have the power to shape our reality and determine whether we approach challenges and trauma with determination or defeat.

Our belief systems absolutely affect how we see the world and what we end up thinking, saying, and doing. When we dive into our beliefs, we start to understand our story about trauma. By paying attention to what we let into our minds and steering our focus, we gain the power to challenge and change those beliefs about ourselves and our experiences. We begin shifting from victim to victor, leaning into the notion that life happens for us. We begin healing.

Beliefs breed action or inaction. Healing is a verb, not a noun.

You are who you think you are and will achieve what you believe.

The jets stopped. Apparently, it was time to get my pruney fingers out of the water.

CHAPTER 14

Action

"For all sad words of tongue and pen, the saddest are these, 'it might have been'... "The journey of a thousand miles must begin with a single step."
—Maud Muller

The sun was peeking through the clouds high in the sky, casting different shades over the rugged landscape of New Zealand. As we gazed out at the breathtaking view before us, I couldn't help but marvel at the striking contrast between lush greenery spreading throughout the rocky ridges and the shimmering aqua blue waters of the river below.

Kyle and I stood near the edge of the building, overlooking the Kawarau Bridge, a rust-colored iron structure decorated with ropes dangling at various intervals to show its charm. We were about to embark on an adventure unlike any other: bungee jumping. Even though this time of year is warm, we were required to dress "appropriately." With my heart already pounding in my chest, I felt a mix of enthusiasm and anxiety.

Despite having pre-registered online, we still had to check in at the counter and sign an additional waiver. "So, I sign my life away here?" I joked with the young man behind the counter, trying to lighten the mood.

"Yep, I guess so," he replied with a grin, his eyes vibrant with amusement as he handed me the paperwork. His low-key laugh added to the casual-thrilling atmosphere of the place.

"Is this your first time bungee jumping?" he asked, his tone friendly and reassuring.

"Yes, I believe so for both of us," I replied, passing the signed forms back to him.

"Well, this will be a great experience. Trust me, you have nothing to worry about," he reassured us with genuine warmth in his voice.

"Okay, thank you," I replied, feeling a mix of "but did you die" slogan assurance as we walked away with our assigned numbers in hand. These numbers would determine the order in which everyone would take the plunge.

"Be sure to stop back and see me afterwards," he shouted.

Kyle and I waved like kids in a candy store, eager to get back outside.

As we approached the Bungy Pod, upbeat music filled the air, booming throughout the structure and infusing it with energy. The lively tunes added to the pulsating excitement, setting the stage for the adrenaline-pumping experience that awaited bystanders watching on deck or those of us preparing to take the leap of faith.

I couldn't shake the nervous fluttering in my stomach, even though this was my idea after all. The thought of throwing myself off the edge of the bridge and into the unknown sounded like a good idea a few days ago. I knew, despite the fear I now felt, I was not going to let it hold me back. If anything, this was my moment of truth, an opportunity to let go of things holding me back – a chance to take some power back.

Of course, my number was called first. Hubby and I walked together over to the loading zone. "Alright babe, we're in this together," he squeezed my hand reassuringly.

I offered him a weak smile and a wink. But as the moment of truth drew near, I found myself still hesitating. *Why the heck am I so nervous? I'm being ridiculous,* I thought to myself. I have jumped out of airplanes – multiple times before.

What if something went wrong? What if the cord snapped, sending me plummeting into the cool waters below?

"Look at that couple," he said, pointing to an elderly pair who were wet and must have been nearing eighty years old.

"Oh yes, they are locals and come here often," one of the employees stated.

Crouching down, I carefully crossed my way between bridge sections, the metallic structure vibrating beneath my touch. Here, two employees awaited, their expert hands ready to guide me through the final stages of preparation. I stepped into a harness that snugly caressed my butt cheeks, providing a sense of security. Looking below at the flowing water, "I'm sure this feels much higher than it actually is," I thought out loud.

With a deep breath, I settled onto the second platform. A rush of anticipation was coursing through my veins. With practiced precision, the employees worked quickly to secure my feet into the bungee cord, double-checking each buckle and strap to ensure that everything was in place. With each tug of the buckle, I grew more and more aware of the magnitude of what I was about to do.

I was unsure if I was truly ready to take the plunge and embrace the unknown. I hesitated for just a moment, with the thought of releasing myself – from myself.

"I-I don't know if I can do this," I stammered, my voice trembling with uncertainty.

"Come on, Stephanie! You got this!" the cute bungee jumping instructor called out.

Taking tentative, tiny steps towards the edge of the platform, my heart was now in my throat. I felt like I was walking the plank. I peered over and glanced down again at the beautiful river below. "Get out of your own damn way, Stephanie."

The male instructor placed a reassuring hand on my shoulder, his eyes filled with understanding. "It's okay to be scared," he said calmly. "But sometimes, you just have to go for it and take that first step, even if it's a small one."

With his words in my mind, I summoned the courage within me. Deliberately, cautiously, I continued tiptoeing forward, my left hand gripping the side ledge firmly. My toes were curled over in my shoes. And although smiling, my entire body raced with fear. Just as I reached the edge, the instructor had one last comment.

"Come on, Wonder-Woman! You're not afraid of a little dip in the water, are you?" he asked humorously.

His words caught me off guard, but I couldn't help but laugh. Kyle must have told him my secret. He then pointed directly out in front of me, "smile and wave," as a small drone buzzed by overhead. I gave the "gnarly" hand signal and stuck out my tongue.

Now I just needed to let go. And by let go, I mean jump!

"You got this, Steph!" Kyle called out with pride from the side viewing area. I also waved to him for a second photo opp.

Releasing my left hand and knees shaking, I opened my chest and spread my wings.

"Alright, I'm going to count down, and you're going to jump! 5, 4, 3, 2, 1."

With one final glance at the horizon, I took a leap of faith, launching myself off the ledge and into the open air.

I was flying.

For a moment, I felt weightless.

As the wind whipped past my ears, I felt a sense of freedom unlike anything before.

I let out a triumphant whoop, my heart soaring with joy. Then for a split second, everything was silent.

I think I blacked out.

The second bounce jolted me back to reality. Just before touching the cool water below, I remember thinking, What a rush! With a huge grin plastered on my face. It felt like a rebirth, like I was emerging anew.

As I hung there like a baby on a bungee umbilical cord, a bright yellow raft with two guys made its way over to catch me. They undid the straps, and I dropped into the boat, feeling more alive than ever before.

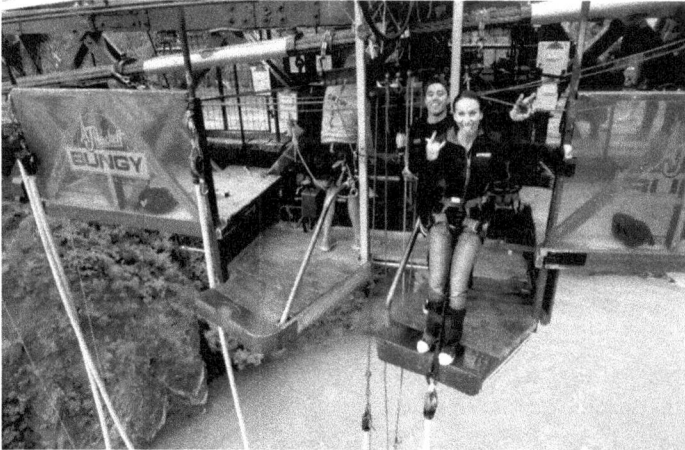

Many of us have fallen for the idea that we have to wait until we feel completely ready before tackling tough challenges. I'll admit, I've bought into that myth myself.

We're led to believe that someday we'll magically have all the confidence we need to take on something new, make a change, or do the scary thing. But here's the reality: our brains aren't wired that way. Instead, they're wired to keep us safe, to steer us away from discomfort or anything that might seem risky.

I've learned that it's natural to never feel fully ready – whether it's to bungee jump off a bridge or navigate the journey of healing. I've also learned that what's important is taking imperfect action – diving in even when we're not completely sure of ourselves. We often build up the first step so much in our minds, but once it's over, we realize how easy it was to let go.

Self-awareness and exploring our belief systems are essential mindsets, but giving ourselves permission is the first *imperfect* action we should take in order to begin healing. Many of us struggle to grant ourselves permission, or the *freedom* to be who we truly want to be and to make our own conscious decisions.

Often, we leave our beliefs unexamined and let our trauma define us as victims. Letting go of these expectations from past trauma sets us up for success, allowing us to create a life based on accepting where we are, who we truly are, and what we genuinely want.

Beginning or continuing a healing journey through imperfect action means embracing progress over perfection and taking mini, manageable steps forward. The biggest hurdle is getting out of our own way! And, you've already taken some action. You are reading this book (thank you)!

Reflecting on that dark chapter of my life, I realized that the first steps toward healing didn't look like a grand transformation; they were small but meaningful pivots. After the sexual assault, I eventually stopped drinking and left behind basketball, both of which had become tangled with memories I wanted to escape. I needed a new direction, something that wasn't about dulling the pain but about finding strength.

That's when pole vaulting found me – a seemingly unlikely passion that catapulted me into college and a new chapter, one where I could redefine love, sex, and most importantly, myself.

It became my daily focus, one step at a time. Shifting my energy from what had hurt me to something that could build me up, gave me the strength I needed.

With every jump, I wasn't just clearing a bar – I was finding a way to rise above the trauma.

The daily work of living is the actual work of healing.

Healing happens in the daily choices we make to live fully in the present, not in what could or *should* have been.

It's about embracing imperfect action, pausing when needed, and shaping a life with intention – moment by moment.

It might mean going for a short walk in the sunshine, spending a quiet moment in gratitude, or simply taking deep breaths to center yourself. It could be choosing to eat a healthy meal, reaching out to a friend for support, allowing yourself to rest when you need it, or even taking on a new hobby like pole-vaulting.

For some, it means surrounding ourselves with the people and experiences that bring joy and growth, or choosing to release the anger and expectations to embrace what has happened *for* us.

These small, intentional acts breathe life into our healing journey, reminding us that every step forward, no matter how small, is a step toward wholeness.

I have redefined what healing means in my life, and it's not a destination.

My friend, I give you and I both permission – permission to act, to take imperfect action, and to make mistakes while we learn from them along the way.

CHAPTER 15

Service

"Service to others is the rent you pay for your room here on Earth." —Muhammad Ali

---

The air is thick with disinfectant, tinged with the lingering smell of fear and desperation. As I walk through the eroded, squeaky door into the cool, windowless room filled with rows of metal cages, I'm met with eyes full of uncertainty and anxiety.

Each animal here carries a story of abandonment, neglect, or cruelty, and every one of them longs for a home – a place to feel safe and loved.

The reality of humane euthanasia looms over staff and volunteers alike. With limited resources and an overwhelming tide of pet overpopulation, tough decisions are often unavoidable. But even in the midst of these harsh realities, there are stories that remind us why community service and volunteering matter – stories of hope, healing, and resilience.

Take Rainbow, for example. This tiny cream-and-white kitten arrived on a frigid day in late November. He was only four months old and had been found huddled under someone's porch, shivering and desperate for warmth and protection. Thankfully, the homeowners were able to coax him into a carrier and bring him to the shelter. Rainbow was so terrified that staff placed him in a quiet space to help him feel safe. But when they were finally able to examine him, their hearts sank. Rainbow's tail had been cut off, and what remained had been degloved all the way to his spine. A devastating injury like this can be life-threatening. If damage reaches the spinal nerves, it can cause permanent incontinence, leaving a kitten unable to control his bladder or bowels.

Luckily, after a thorough evaluation, staff confirmed that Rainbow hadn't suffered permanent nerve damage. He would need surgery to repair his stump, but he had a chance. Despite his trauma, Rainbow displayed a fierce will to survive. With patience and care, this little warrior healed and found his forever home.

But not all cats do.

Sometimes, animals arrive so deeply traumatized that it's hard to know if they can ever "recover." Gabby was one of those dogs. The moment she entered the shelter, it was clear her past had been filled with torment and abuse. Her entire body trembled with fear. She refused to walk, curling up into a tiny, quivering ball anytime someone approached. Staff had to carry her everywhere – even outside to go to the bathroom. The slightest touch made her defecate in terror. Our hearts crumbled seeing the depths of her pain, wondering if we could ever show her that not all humans were the enemy.

Knowing the noise and commotion in the dog kennel area would overwhelm her, the staff gave Gabby a quiet space in the front office. Staff and volunteers spent countless hours sitting on the floor beside her, gently stroking her and speaking in low, calm voices. At first, Gabby lay frozen in fear, cowering in the corner. But over time, she started poking her nose out, little by little, curious but cautious. One day at a time, Gabby began trusting the world around her again. Eventually, she found a loving forever home.

But not all dogs do.

Every week, I volunteer at the local animal shelter, surrounded by the heart-wrenching sounds of dogs barking and crying, critters scurrying about their cages, and cats meowing desperately to get out from behind their bars.

The shelter is not a peaceful sanctuary, but rather what I believe to be a stark reminder of the failures of humanity.

Shelters like this one exist because we, as a society, have not adequately cared for these animals. For many of them, this is their last resort, their final hope for a second, or even a third chance at life.

I do my part – and it has helped in many ways.

One particular afternoon, the kennel manager called out to me as soon as I walked in for my cat socialization volunteer shift. "I shouldn't even tell you this," she said with a knowing smile. "You have to see the new kitty that came in last week. I think you are going to love him."

She led me into the "staff only" room where animal intake is completed. This also happens to be the shared space for laundry and humane euthanasia.

On the far wall was a cage where a small, 9 month old ragdoll mix cat named Cosmo sat huddled in the corner near his tiny metal litter box. His large, expressive blue eyes were filled with confusion and hope.

"What!? Look at this adorable boy with the little gray mustache-like spot near his nose and whiskers. How did he get here?" I asked, even though it broke my heart to learn the truth, every single time.

"His previous owner surrendered him due to landlord issues," the manager explained. "I doubt it. She simply didn't want him – and he's so sweet. Shhhhhh. I'm not supposed to allow him out yet, but I'll let you take him for a few minutes."

I knelt down and gently opened the cage door. "Hey there, Cosmo, you handsome boy," I whispered. As I extended my hands, he leaned in with a soft 'hello' purr, his soft, warm head pressing securely against my hand. With an intense, affectionate motion, he nudged his head up and down, his whiskers brushing against my fingers.

"You're safe here, buddy," I continued, interpreting his now-loud meows as a dialogue of mutual understanding. "We've both been through a lot, haven't we?"

Walking into the social room with him, I sat Cosmo down and laid on the old, cold, chipping cement floor. Cosmo strutted over to my chest and flopped over, his forehead making contact with a loving push against my cheek. His white fur and fuzzy tail on my face had me laughing. "I know honey, I love you too already." Being present with animals helps me heal just as much as it helps them.

Cosmo was my kitty! There was no denying it.

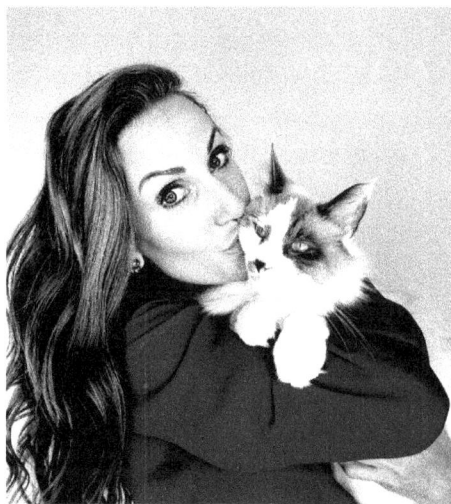

It took under two minutes to form an unconditional bond. "Daddy's going to be jealous. We should send him a quick video. What do you think?" I was no novice at talking to animals.

Kyle of course was onboard with adopting him. "What's one more kitty?" We laughed.

Cosmo's story, along with Rainbow and Gabby, mirrored my own in so many ways. Just as they had been displaced and found themselves in a vulnerable position, I too had felt powerless and voiceless at various points in my life. But while helping them, and the countless other animals that come through the shelter doors every year, I was finding a way to use my reclaimed voice and power.

I believe that giving is living!

And my instant connection with Cosmo – my experience of finding safety and trust through service, has become a pillar of my life and healing journey.

The act of giving back, of being present for these vulnerable creatures, has provided me with a profound sense of purpose and inspiration. When I first began volunteering, sure, I was seeking a way to cope with my own feelings of guilt. But more importantly, I had been blessed with the gift of schedule flexibility and desired to be a part of something bigger than myself.

Supporting animals like Cosmo, Rainbow, Gabby and their thousands of furry friends who have been abandoned or mistreated, provides hope for many to bounce back from trauma and find triumph.

A significant part of healing is recognizing that what happens *for* us can also be used as fuel to help others. This intentional, systemic shift in perspective is about making the conscious choice every day to express gratitude and give back, whether to ourselves or others.

Remember when I said, *rarely do we heal by accident*? Healing is not a passive process; but does require active engagement and commitment to small, daily habits that foster a sense of purpose and connection to ourselves and the world.

Research consistently shows that helping others can significantly improve our mental health.

Since the pandemic in 2020, it seems many individuals are struggling now more than ever. I have found that giving back and expressing gratitude can reduce fear and grief, while increasing feelings of social connectedness and overall well-being.

Every time I kneel down to comfort a frightened cat or help an excited dog find a new home; I am reminded of my own journey. These acts of service are not just about the animals; they are about healing my own bullshit, too.

By giving my time, energy and love, I am, in a way, giving back to myself.

Giving back has taught me that healing and service go hand in hand. The more I give, the more I heal, and the more I heal, the more I become my true, authentic self.

Giving is living!

For me, volunteering has been more than just a therapeutic activity; it has been a life raft.

Service is not what I do, it's who I am!

By using our experiences to help others, we transform our pain into purpose. We become active participants in our own healing and in the healing of those around us.

The act of serving others, even when we are going through difficult times, reinforces the idea that we are all connected and that our actions create lasting ripple effects.

That is the power of service.

CHAPTER 16

Lighthouses

"Only when we're brave enough to explore the darkness will we discover the infinite power of our light." —Brene Brown

---

For the longest time, I blamed my parents and parental role models for "destroying" me. Reflecting back to childhood and the stories I've shared, my early fears of rejection and urge for validation and voice became the causation of my watered down self-worth issues that emerged in adulthood.

I believed I wasn't good enough, not deserving of a spectacular life. But my mindset changed.

Change your story. Change your life.

I used to think trauma healing was a subtractive process – shedding everything that didn't serve my sanity or bring genuine joy and fulfillment to my life. It meant removing the murky parts I didn't want others to see or understand.

But the more I tried to strip away, the shittier I felt. Turns out, bypassing pieces of who I am, is a game I'd never win.

Many of us tiptoe around our own psyche, but every experience – whether a major event or a tiny, unnoticed wound – resides within us like hidden beacons waiting to shine. Even the stuff we try to sweep under the mental rug becomes part of our identity, influencing us whether we like it or not.

For too long, my vessel was shrouded in fog. I felt disconnected from myself and my humanness.

The day I resigned, hitting "enter" on my keyboard was like pressing the reset button. I wrote down the following in my journal: "Who do you want to be? Take an honest inventory..."

Life puts us in a position for action – messy action.

Action is energy. Everything in life is energy.

Thank you Energy.

Thank you Action.

And thank you crappy...trauma. Gratitude.

Expressing gratitude has helped shift my mindset. Yeah, I still think cat poop on my ex-coworker's porch is funny. But I'm no longer angry.

In fact, I'm grateful. I'm grateful for the gift of schedule flexibility and something new. Ever notice how each day typically starts in the dark? So why are we afraid to use our dark side for new beginnings?

Slowly I began realizing that the dark parts of my life were not burdens to discard. Their presence was not accidental; they were reminders of my humanity and capacity to experience all emotions.

Just as we can't appreciate the warmth of the sun without knowing the chill of the night, we can't truly feel joy without having known sorrow, or passion without experiencing pain. It's the contrast between light and dark that deepens our understanding and appreciation of both.

In my journal, I also wrote: "every new day comes with a new opportunity to define what 'enough' means to me." On the back of the page, I continued to scribble, "life feels short and I want to be uplifted, colorful, empowered in my own skin and unapologetic AF about it!"

Skipping a line on the page, I continued writing, "I want to be love and light." This sentence had been crossed out, and below in caps, I wrote:

"I AM LOVE AND LIGHT!"

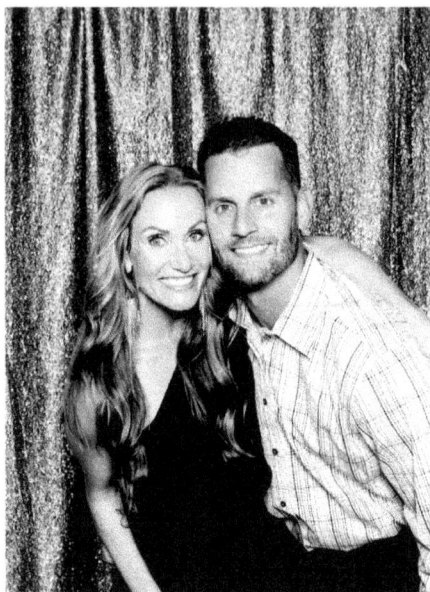

Every experience has led me to where I am now, quite literally writing this book.

I needed those times that knocked me flat on my ass just as much as I needed those times of feeling on top of the world. I don't regret any of it.

Without the dysfunction, I wouldn't have the ambitions that drive me. I wouldn't be the strong woman I am today. Without the trauma, I wouldn't have built the muscle to want more, to be more and to give more.

Without the darkness, I wouldn't be the light.

I learned to wade through what I didn't want to truly appreciate and embrace the clear waters of what I unequivocally deserve. Sometimes, the moments you wish you could delete from your life are the very ones that turned you into the badass you are today.

My parents and parental figures did not destroy me. They unknowingly gifted me with an insatiable thirst and an unstoppable determination I never asked for.

My journey from trauma to triumph has been mostly a process of surrender; a shift in perspective towards my experiences.

Surrendering is not a subtractive process, or about denying the past; it's about embracing every part of ourselves. What once seemed like burdens become badges of honor, beacons of hope and reminders of the strength within us.

As I continue my journey, I'm growing, thriving, and learning to evaluate myself more accurately. It's in this brave act of self-confrontation, when I "SEAS" the day, healing is present.

There's nothing sexier than having the courage to own your truth.

A lighthouse shines brightest against the backdrop of darkness.

By embracing both the light and dark within us, we allow our authentic selves, the messy masterpiece, to illuminate a more empowered path forward.

I am the light – and so are you!

And the darkness is where I learned to shine.

CHAPTER 17

Charting New Horizons

"In the waves of change, we find our true direction."
—Unknown

Never regret a day in your life.

Good days give you happiness. Bad days give you experiences.

The worst days give you lessons. The best days give you memories.

You cannot have the good without the bad.

The school of life is continually preparing us for the next thing, as we navigate every lesson together. Everyone has their own set of rules, shaped by their personal stories. And we are not supposed to have all the answers. I know I don't!

But what I've learned is this: Life is a gift, always happening *for* us.

This perspective of empowerment allows us to choose the meaning of every experience, even if it takes years to unravel the 'why.' Although life doesn't always hand us reasons wrapped in neat bows; instead, it presents us with moments – both joyous and painful – that we must decipher and make sense of ourselves.

One evening, after a long, emotional day of putting our beloved cat to rest, my husband and I stopped at the bar for our usual Old Fashioned. The familiar taste offered a small comfort among our shared grief. We quickly returned home to our cozy living room, wrapped ourselves in blankets, and turned on the TV for some background noise to drown out my sobbing.

"Babe," I began, looking into his eyes, "I'm super sad right now. And also so grateful for everything we've been through together. Every challenge, every trip... it's all shaped us into the couple we are today."

He squeezed my hand, his eyes reflecting a mix of sorrow and love. "Yeah, me too. We've been through a lot these past few years."

"She was always there for me," I said, my voice trembling. "Through so much...Malibu was my everything."

He nodded, his grip on my hand tightening. "She was special. Always knew when you needed her. Mali was loved – and she will be missed."

"I know we've been through worse, but my heart feels broken." I continued. "Thank you for being here."

"We've supported each other through so much shit," I continued. "And each time, we've come out stronger."

"I hurt too. It sucks." He sighed, his eyes distant for a moment. "Malibu will always be with us. She lived a great life and will watch over us from across the rainbow bridge."

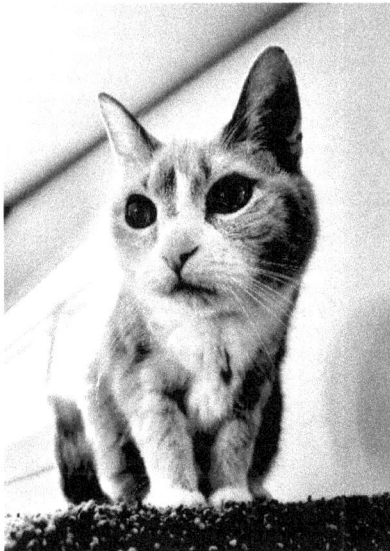

"Yeah," I said, my voice breaking slightly. "I just hope she knew how much she meant to me...to us. I just don't understand death..."

"Yeah," he said quietly. "We will figure it out – like we always do – one step, one day at a time."

"I love you," I whispered.

"I love me too," he said with a smirk.

He always has a way of lightening the mood. Afterall, humor is why I married the man. Haha. I hope he reads this part.

True healing from any trauma isn't a destination, it's a continuous voyage. Every day, we navigate through the choppy waters of past and present, working to integrate our experiences into the DNA of who we are.

I learned healing is an active, daily commitment. Healing is waking up each day and choosing to sail forward, even when we'd much rather hit the snooze button a few times.

In my journey, I've aligned myself with the acronym "SEAS" – Self-Awareness, Exploring Belief Systems, Action, and Service. These principles guide me through the storms and the stillness, ensuring that I steer my life with courage, intention, and purpose. They remind me to live authentically, to reject society's expectations, and to build a life that resonates with my true self – my true North.

I hope my words inspire you to take back your joy and self-worth. I hope you too, use your voice to illuminate what's been buried in the darkness.

Self-Awareness keeps us grounded, exploring our belief systems broadens our horizons, taking action propels us forward, and service to others connects us to the world. By embracing these principles, we can live lives of depth and meaning.

Let your life be a testament to the power of resilience and the beauty of imperfection.

Embrace it all, for our darkest moments set the stage for our greatest revelations – our naked truths.

Sail confidently into the unknown, trusting that you have the strength to weather any storm and the wisdom to create meaning through the waters of existence.

"SEAS" the day, every day, and let your journey inspire others to do the same.

The truth is:

- The same storm that shakes us to our core, also harbors the guiding currents toward a clearer shore.
- Anchors, both visible and invisible, have the strength to pull us down or keep us stagnant unless we choose to disrupt their hold on us.
- Your life is your story. Write it well. Edit it often.
- We must be grateful for closed doors, bad vibes, and stuff that falls apart. It's universal protection from people, places and things that are no longer in alignment with your soul. Sometimes it's not what we want, but what we need.
- Encouraging someone to be entirely themselves is the loudest way to love them.
- Only when we seek to understand ourselves, can we truly focus our efforts on what requires attention and healing.
- You are who you think you are and will achieve what you believe.
- Life. The whole damn thing is about decisions. Every path you take leads to another choice. And some choices will change everything.

- Healing is a verb, not a noun.
- Small steps still move you forward.
- By using our experiences to help others, we transform our pain into purpose.
- The darkness is where we learn to shine.

In the lush ocean of life, here I thought I was drowning. But really, I was learning to swim all along.

And that's my **naked truth!**

Epilogue

"It is good to have an end to journey toward; but it is the journey that matters, in the end."
—Ernest Hemingway

We are human. We are flawed. We are messy. We are self-fish. We are beautiful.

And we all have a story to share.

Today, someone asked what inspires me. After a pause, I replied, "People that have experienced great setbacks in their life, but still find the courage to carry on."

Not only does this feel inspiring, it fuels me with the fight to wake up each morning and "SEAS" the day.

We can learn to love ourselves through both the good times and bad. In fact, I believe we should love ourselves even more during times of trauma, because those experiences are not distractions from life – they are life.

Life happens for us!

One day, you will tell people how you pulled yourself out of the ocean when you could not even swim.

I hope when I'm long gone, people will say that I made an impact.

SEASide Station

It seems overwhelming to leave what you know behind and start forward on an uncharted path. If you could stay with me this far on my journey, I believe you are powerful enough to brave the SEAS and start your journey too.

Here are some activities and reflection prompts to help.

Self-Awareness:

- Check out this Youtube video:
  https://www.youtube.com/watch?v=IGQmdoK_ZfY

Body Scan Exercises

- A practice that helps you connect with your emotions and physiology. By systematically focusing on sensations throughout your body, you become more aware of physical tension and can eventually release it. Take notice in various environments. Try this around groups of friends and family. Or, go for a walk outside and notice.

Gratitude Exercises

- Write down five to ten things you are grateful for in the morning or before bed. This can help you focus on what is working and ground yourself.

Exploring Belief Systems:

Sticky Note Self-Talk

- Write three to five positive affirmations on sticky notes. Post them on your bathroom mirror. Read them every morning. Ex. I am worthy. I am a published author, etc. Think-speak-believe them into existence.

Journaling

- Writing down your thoughts and feelings in a journal can help you identify recurring patterns and themes in your thinking. By reflecting on your experiences and the words you use to describe them, you can gain insight into the underlying beliefs that shape your worldview.

Mindfulness Practices

- https://www.mindful.org/practice-art-being-present/ Engaging in mindfulness meditation or other mindfulness techniques can help you observe your thoughts without judgment. By paying attention to the words and phrases that arise in your mind, you can become more aware of the beliefs that influence your thinking and behavior.

Therapy or Counseling

- Working with a therapist or counselor can provide a supportive environment for exploring and challenging your beliefs. Through guided discussion and reflection, you can uncover the underlying beliefs that drive your thoughts and actions, and work towards creating more empowering beliefs.

Seeking Feedback

- Asking trusted friends, family members, or colleagues for feedback on your words and behavior can provide valuable insights into your belief systems. Others may notice patterns or themes in your communication that you may not be aware of, helping you gain a deeper understanding of your beliefs.

Reading and Self-study

- Engaging in reading and self-study on topics related to psychology, personal development, and emotional intelligence can broaden your perspective and provide new insights into your own beliefs. By learning about different theories and perspectives, you can challenge and expand your understanding of yourself and the world around you.

Action:

"Five Senses" Exercise

- Actively noticing sights, sounds, smells, tastes, and textures around you helps to ground you in the present moment, reducing distractions and allowing for focused action.

Pray and Meditate

- Focus on your breath and present sensations, and observe your thoughts and feelings without judgment.
- Practice hearing the voice of the universe and WRITE it down. Always have a pen and journal.
  - Jim Rohn – "A life worth living is a life worth recording" – He said to keep a journal and it serves like a GPS.

Mindful Walking

- Paying close attention to the physical sensations of walking, like the movement of your feet and the rhythm of your steps, can help you recenter yourself.

Read

- Similar to the aforementioned. Learn to invest in yourself.

Listen to Audio Messages

- Use drive time to learn and grow. Turn your car into your classroom.
- Use a sticky note that says, "push play" for when you get ready in the morning.

Service:

Give Back - We Rise by Lifting Others

- Find ways to give back within your local community. Connect with your local Chamber to learn about opportunities.
- Volunteer for a local organization. What are you passionate about?
- Rather than mundane birthday or holiday gifts, ask for monetary donations for a local charity of choice.
- Collect food, clothing or other supplies for a non-profit organization in need.

Did you have any moments of clarity or any "aha" moments in this book? I'd be so grateful if you would leave a quick review on Amazon. It takes less than two minutes and goes a long way in helping others navigate their own trauma.

Thank you for spreading the word!

Follow Stephanie Kraemer:

Facebook: https://www.facebook.com/stephanie.pavletich
Instagram: @stephaniejkraemer

About the Author

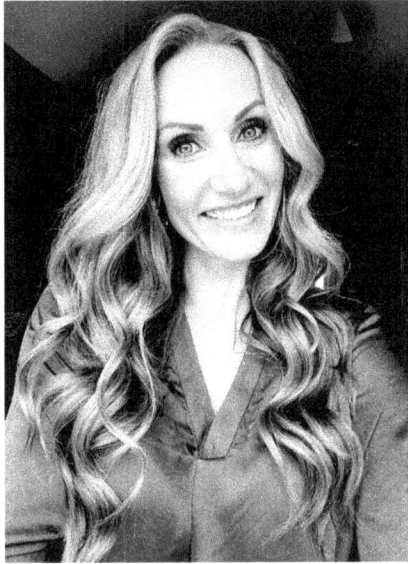

Stephanie Kraemer is an author, speaker, and animal ambassador dedicated to empowering individuals to live a life of authenticity and service. With a passion for education, Stephanie has inspired countless people to become the heroes of their own stories through her unique approach to self-discovery, SEAS the day. Her sassy style and heartfelt wisdom make her a sought-after speaker and a beloved figure in her community. After quitting her corporate job to pursue a freelance life, her animal advocacy efforts shine through her volunteer work with local shelters and her partnership with WMTV15, inspiring the adoption of animals in need. Stephanie lives in Wisconsin with her husband and shit load of adorable fur babies.

Acknowledgements

"The sea drives truth into a man like salt."
—Hilaire Belloc

One of the most beautiful things about being a writer is that you cannot do it alone.

This book has been a labor of love, and I'd like to start by thanking my awesome husband, Kyle. From support to quit the bullshit to early draft reads, to providing valuable feedback and time to heal. He was as important to this book getting written as I was. Thank you so much, babe.

Enormous thanks to everyone at She Rises Studios; Angie and Katrina, my editors; and the greatest graphic design team I could ever imagine.

Thanks to everyone in the Punchy Book Program; my group members and incredible accountability buddy, April.

Additionally, I want to thank:

My mom and dad, for creating me.

My friend Lisa for beta reading and editing. You are an amazing human.

My best friends Liz and Shanna.

My hairdresser and therapist, Lauren.

I want to thank EVERYONE who has inspired me, ever said anything positive to me, or taught me something. I heard it all, and it meant the world.

And most of all, thank you readers for the opportunity to express my vulnerability. We all have a story – now go share yours!

www.ingramcontent.com/pod-product-compliance
Lightning Source LLC
Chambersburg PA
CBHW060240030426

42335CB00014B/1544